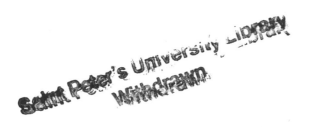

"WE HAVE
A DONOR"

"WE HAVE A DONOR"

The Bold New World
of Organ Transplanting

MARK DOWIE

ST. MARTIN'S PRESS
NEW YORK

For
Wendy

Design by Robert Bull Design.

Library of Congress Cataloging-in-Publication Data

Dowie, Mark.
    We have a donor : the bold new world of organ transplanting / Mark Dowie.
        p.   cm.
    ISBN 0-312-02316-2
    1. Transplantation of organs, tissues, etc.—Moral and ethical aspects.   2. Transplantation of organs, tissues, etc.—Economic aspects.   I. Title.
RD120.7.D69   1988
617'.95—dc19   88-17650

First Edition

10 9 8 7 6 5 4 3 2 1

CONTENTS

ACKNOWLEDGMENTS

While working on this book, I basked in the warmth, friendship, support, and hospitality of many people, all of whom inspired me, many of whose ideas I borrowed, and most of whom will remain lifelong friends.

Of the surgeons who took moments or hours from their incredible schedules to explain the arcane secrets of their technology, none was more generous than Nicholas Feduska at the University of California, San Francisco. Rarely is an author granted the privilege of such scrutiny. I watched him operate, he took me on rounds, I observed him counseling the families of very sick people, he allowed me to witness the recipient selection process, he spent hours on the phone defining terms, describing techniques, explaining policies. Nick, I couldn't have done this without your patience and generosity.

Other physicians who contributed generously of their time and research include Felix Rapaport, John Najarian, Larry Pitts, Sir Roy Calne, Stuart Jamieson, Jean Hamburger, Francis Moore, Paul Byrne, Jean Dausset, Nancy Ascher, Henri Kreis, Gary Friedlaender, René Küss, Ronald Cranford, Richard Simmons, Oscar Salvatierra, Jr., Leonard Bailey, Keith Reemtsma, Sir Peter Medawar, Marvin Garovoy, Thomas Starzl, Christian Cabrol, John Brems, and Leo J. P. Clark.

To health professionals Amy Peele, Ron Dreffer, Lisa Tulman, Robert Capito, Carol Fink, Tom Chakurda, Leslee Boyd, Jerold Mande, Arthur Caplan, and Arthur Harrel, thanks for answering all my questions.

The assistance and hospitality of Henry Spira, Charles Mann, Gwenda Blair, Sophie Craighead, Shoon Murray, Mark Hertsgaard, Yvonne Lembi, Pierre Plousseau, Peter Schneider, Mark Lebarle, Sudi Schneider, Catherine David, Isi Beller, and the Center for Investigative Reporting were indispensable.

And without support from the Engelhard Foundation, Naneen Karraker, George Klingelhoffer, the Fund for Investigative Journalism, Alvin Duskin, and Stanley Sheinbaum, this would have been a very thin book indeed.

Journalistic apologies to David Zinman, Andrew Schneider, and all other reporters whose quotes I lifted without each time attributing their journals. I did so with the philosophical premise that the quotes were given by the original sources to the public at large, not just to the *Pittsburgh Press*, *New York Newsday*, or the *Times*.

And finally, I want to thank my editors at St. Martin's Press: Felicia Eth, who guided the project into existence, and Michael Sagalyn, who made it sing.

INTRODUCTION

Though a simple operative curiosity today,
the transplant of a gland may perhaps someday have
a practical application.

ALEXIS CARREL
Nobel Laureate
1901

The transfer of body parts from one human being to another, written off by great medical thinkers of the 1940s and 1950s as eccentric, evolved in the second half of this century from a rare curiosity to a recognized treatment. Organ and tissue transplants are now performed routinely in the major medical centers of Europe and North America. Surgeons in the United States transplanted almost 15,000 vital organs in 1987.

Yet, in a technical sense, transplantation remains in its infancy. It is about where Henry Ford was when he began to mass-produce the Model T—at that critical, exciting point in the history of any new product when R&D has given an enterprise enough technology to begin production.

Within the next five years the art of transplantation will advance as far as it has in the past thirty. And as it does, just as easily as it evolved from experiment to specialty, it will grow to become a full-scale medical industry, one that will affect not only the selective treatment of organ failure but, ultimately, the way we attack many other diseases.

At this very moment there are 90,000 Americans on dialysis who could benefit from a new kidney. Every year an estimated 15,000 die who could have been saved by a new heart. Add thousands more who have been told they need livers, pancreases, middle ears, corneas, skin, bone, bone marrow, and joints, and one has enough demand to nourish any venture for years to come. Supply, however, remains limited, partly because of the hesitancy of people to donate their own or loved ones' organs after death, and partly because of the reluctance of healthcare professionals to ask for them.

Despite the persistent shortage of organs, there is already a transplant unit in or near every major city and at almost every state university in the United States and medical school in Europe, each with a long list of slowly dying patients who have watched the miracle of transplantation played out before them on the morning news and believe it can work for them. And despite the scarcity, there are few hospitals of any size on either continent that are not discussing the possibility of adding transplantation to their surgical services.

On drawing boards in Pittsburgh, Pennsylvania, and Paris, France, are vast medical centers that will do little else but replace worn and diseased organs and tissues. A French physician shows off plans for the center where he hopes one day to practice his specialty, and calmly predicts that before the end of the century more than half the major surgical operations in the Western world will involve the replacement of organs and other body parts. Professional hype? Maybe. Perhaps mere wishful thinking. It really doesn't matter. The dream is alive and expansion is under way. The impact of organ transplantation on medicine, health policy, and the biological sciences is only beginning to be felt. And as it becomes more successful, demand for the service will continue to escalate.

In some respects this story is as old as medicine. Long before the earliest healers knew what caused the simplest diseases, physicians were trying to replace limbs and organs that had failed or fallen from their fellow human beings. Until very recently, most attempts were met with sad, even tragic, failure. Only within the last ten years have these attempts begun to work well enough for medical practitioners and health planners to feel comfortable using the word "treatment" instead of "experiment" when speaking of tissue and organ transplantation.

Research, not practice, has been the driving force of organ transplantation, as it must be in any high-technology venture. That won't change. The illusive quest for induced tolerance of foreign tissue presses on. In the meantime, drugs are developed to contain the immune response, organs are preserved for longer and longer periods, brain-dead cadavers are kept "reanimated" for days, new grafts are perfected (pancreases, lungs, intestines, thymus glands, hands, testes, fetal tissue, and, if not brains, brain cells), bionics are advanced, and subhuman primates are raised to provide organs for humans.

All of it, of course, is merely a temporary stage of medical development that awaits the day when either we find the cure for end-stage organ diseases or "designer" organs are produced on command from healthy cells implanted in the body. In the meantime, the medical, legal, and religious communities must deal with the moral and ethical challenges brought to them by contemporary transplanters. Their dilemmas are inescapable.

This week Norman Shumway, chief of heart transplantation at Stanford University, has to decide who, from his long list of waiting patients, gets a donor heart that turns up with barely a moment's notice. As he ponders his decision, he will know that one, maybe two, of the patients not selected will die before the next heart arrives.

John Najarian, chief of surgery at the University of Minnesota (Minneapolis), scans his liver ward and decides whether to transplant a patient on the verge of death or the one down the hall, less sick and therefore less likely to waste the scarce and precious organ.

Tom Starzl, the University of Pittsburgh's pioneer transplanter, decides whether to give another liver to a patient who has already rejected two or to give the new organ to a better-matched patient waiting for his first. Sir Roy Calne, Starzl's friend and co-mentor in Cambridge, England, agonizes over whether to replace a cirrhotic liver in an alcoholic. And Oscar Salvatierra, Jr., head of transplantation at the University of California, San Francisco, defends his controversial practice of removing kidneys from living donors, while raising doubts about whether David Sutherland should do the same thing with a pancreas in Minnesota.

Meanwhile, bone marrow transplanter Robert Gale of UCLA deliberates with his staff and administration over the politically explosive question of whether or not to transplant liver cells, brain cells, and other tissues from aborted fetuses. The National Association of Transplant Coordinators debates how aggressive to be in organ procurement, the American Association for Tissue Banks struggles with 300 unregulated members who compete vigorously over access to human cadavers, and an unpublicized meeting of pediatric transplanters discusses whether or not the public is ready to accept the harvesting of organs from living babies born with atrophied brains.

The transplanters' ethical plight has already spawned a new subspecialty in the blooming field of bioethics. It has become almost impossible, however, for "transplant ethicists" to keep abreast of the issues. In fact, they can barely contain the community they advise: the surgeons, whose dramatic achievements on the operating table merely embolden the pioneers among them to escalate their pursuit of organs and proceed with the next miracle, challenging, with each new breakthrough, the central tenets of Western medical, legal, religious, and philosophical thought.

The issues emerging from organ transplantation have already reached far beyond medicine. Laws have been passed or amended to redefine death and the rights of survivors. Media managers have altered the way healthcare is covered and reported. And the elders of every great religion in the world have convened to ponder transplantation's impact on their deepest beliefs and dogma.

In a marketplace overflowing with miraculous healing technologies, organ transplantation begins to take its place in line, and is called to question by those who must allocate the ever-shrinking healthcare resources of the wealthiest nations on earth. Even so, there remains a special awe for this bold practice, which offers a last ray of hope to those dying before their time. And why not? It does save some young lives, and we have so much of value to learn from it.

But whether a society, even a wealthy society, should commit massive funds and talent to save a few lives with heroic surgery or invest the same resources in finding ways to cure or eliminate the very diseases and conditions that necessitate the surgery, is a question that will haunt European and American policymakers for years to come. Regardless of their wisdom and practicality, our own appetite for epic rescue and our reverence of technology may well combine to keep organ transplants more alluring than they might otherwise be.

PART ONE

THE TRANSPLANTERS

I*t is impossible to deny the allure of organ transplantation. We watch in absolute amazement as supercooled organs and tissues are sped from city to city in chartered jets and helicopters, from "beating-heart cadavers" in small-town trauma centers to sophisticated urban complexes that form the newest subsidiary of modern medicine—the transplant unit, an institution that is profoundly affecting not only contemporary science and medical philosophy but also our most basic notions about health, healing, life, and death.*

We marvel at heroic, twenty-two-hour operations where "the gift of life" is deftly transferred from the newly dead to the barely living. As we watch, we sense that we are witnessing the very edge of our own existence, and the thrill is not unlike the feeling that comes with the launch of a great space mission or the birth of a child.

Transplantation has already given us a new folklore filled with unforgettable events and heroes. Who of those who were conscious will ever forget the day that Christiaan Barnard removed a living heart from a brain-dead woman and placed it into the chest of a dying Johannesburg grocer; or the morning that little Stormie Jones went home with a new heart and liver, waving good-bye to Tom Starzl, the brilliant surgeon-scientist who saved her life and revolutionized medicine (whether or not for the better remains to be seen)?

With all its miracles and wonders, it is difficult to assess transplantation rationally and acknowledge, along with its promise, its darker aspects—the tremendous expense, the questionable allocation of healthcare resources, and the marginal lives of so many of its survivors. But as with all emerging technologies, closer examination is needed.

CHAPTER 1

JACESOHN AND THE TRANSPLANTERS

It remains now to be seen how society will manage transplantation, the most recent product of its creativity and sponsorship.

THOMAS STARZL, M.D.,
University of Pittsburgh

It begins, as it so often must, with tragedy.

On February 25, 1987, a warm, early spring day in San Francisco, California, a fifteen-year-old Eurasian boy named Jacesohn (pronounced Jason) Walden borrowed a friend's skateboard and headed for his favorite hill. Jacesohn was a good skateboarder, one of the best in the neighborhood, in fact; but this wasn't his skateboard and he wasn't accustomed to its action.

There was no one else on the block when he fell, so it's hard to say what happened; but sometime later that afternoon Jacesohn was found unconscious by a passerby, who called for help. Within minutes an ambulance arrived and rushed him to San Francisco General Hospital, where he regained enough consciousness to respond to simple commands. According to his chart, a CAT scan revealed a "massive epidural hematoma"—a blood clot between his skull and his brain. Again Jacesohn was rushed, this time through the hallways of the hospital to an operating room, where his skull was opened to relieve the pressure that had built on his brain. The surgery went well and for a while his condition improved.

3

Within an hour of Jacesohn's admission, Carol Fink, a psychiatric nurse who specializes in counseling the families of critical care patients, had found his parents, Sam and Virginia Walden. "They were lovely people," Fink remembers. "Sam is from a big warm Italian family, Virginia is Filipino." After days spent with the Waldens, Fink would come to know more about her unconscious patient than she would about his living relatives. "They talked a lot about him," she remembers. "His teen years had been troubled, but these were parents that cared a lot for their children."

In the long days that followed, Jacesohn's condition deteriorated. The wound was deeper than the first CAT scan had indicated. In fact, a closer examination revealed a "progressive cerebral edema"—accumulation of fluids inside the brain. Jacesohn began to present some alarming symptoms. His pupils became fixed and dilated, and would no longer respond to light. He had no reflexes. He could not breathe without a respirator. The line on his electroencephalogram (EEG) screen was flat. And he would not respond to painful stimuli. These were most of the conditions that in California and forty-one other states can now be used, at the discretion of attending physicians, to declare a person brain dead.

No one had given up on Jacesohn, but as the badly wounded youth lay on a respirator in Intensive Care—with heart beating, body warm, and urine passing—subtle changes began to appear in the behavior of hospital staffers around him, including Carol Fink. Drawing from experience, intuition, and some recent training, Fink and her colleagues began to see their deeply comatose patient less as a living human being fighting for his life and more as a dying human being whose organs and tissues might, through transplantation, save others dying elsewhere in the country. The medical care provided Jacesohn himself, of course, remained vigorous. In fact, intensive care nurse Vivian Curd can barely remember fighting harder or longer for a patient in Jacesohn's condition. Everything done for him was part of a desperate attempt to save his life. Yet the early and subtle signs of a new medical procedure, "organ procurement," had commenced.

It began sometime on Sunday morning, March 1, when Jacesohn's attending neurosurgeon, Jonathan Hodes, told Carol Fink he thought the situation was beginning to look hopeless. He was not ready to declare death, he said; more time and more tests were needed. But he was not optimistic.

There were two strong forces at work in Hodes's mind. First and foremost, of course, was the effort to save his patient's life. If that was impossible, Hodes had to be absolutely certain that Jacesohn's condition was hopeless before declaring him dead. The second force involved the lifesaving potential of Jacesohn's organs. Although that was not Hodes's direct responsibility, as a physician he had to be concerned about other patients as well as his own. If he let Jacesohn languish on a respirator until his heart stopped, as it eventually would were he brain dead, his organs would be useless for transplantation.

Shortly after she spoke with Hodes, Carol Fink placed a call to Lisa Tulman, a registered nurse at the University of California hospital, about five miles across San Francisco from General Hospital. Tulman is a coordinator for the UCSF transplant unit. Over the years Tulman and other transplant coordinators in the Bay Area had carefully coached people like Fink to watch for potential organ donors. "Lisa, I may have a donor for you," said Fink. "He's a fifteen-year-old skateboard victim, massive edema, some infarction. Looks bad. He's one hundred fifty-five pounds, blood type A. He's comatose, respirated, and could be declared within forty-eight hours. . . ."

Fink went on to provide the additional information Tulman needed to begin a search of her hospital's long list of patients waiting for new kidneys. In order to target the most appropriate recipient, Tulman would need to know blood type, age, weight, and a few other medical details about the donor. One by one she jotted down the vital numbers as Fink recited them.

Although Jacesohn Walden was legally still alive, the early

stages of San Francisco General Hospital's protocol for organ retrieval had been implemented. And at that point Sam and Virginia Walden had no indication that they might never speak with their son again, or that procedures were under way to harvest his organs.

Before she placed the data Fink had given her into the UCSF computer, Lisa Tulman had some other urgent calls to make. Although UCSF is one of the largest transplant units in the world, at the time it was only transplanting kidneys. Tulman therefore took it upon herself to find heart and liver transplant centers somewhere in the country that might be able to use Jacesohn's other organs.

With Stanford University Hospital in northern California the closest heart transplant unit in Tulman's region, her first call was to Marguerite Brown, Stanford's transplant coordinator. Brown and her world-famous boss, Dr. Norman Shumway, would need to select a recipient for Jacesohn's heart—should he die. The chosen patient could live an hour or more's flying time from the town of Palo Alto, and ideally for the success of a transplant, the recipient needed to be on the operating table and anesthetized when the new heart arrived. The shorter the time Jacesohn's heart existed without blood in it, the better its chances of lasting in a new body.

At the time there was only one hospital that transplanted livers in northern California, where Jacesohn lived. It was in Davis, near Sacramento. Through a nationwide agreement, transplant coordinators try to place organs in the region where they're donated. Tulman called the University of California Davis Medical Center and found that they didn't have a patient who matched Jacesohn's size or blood type. So she called Barbara Nuesse, a coordinator at the Regional Organ Procurement Agency in Los Angeles, whose job is to locate and procure kidneys, hearts, livers, and pancreases for patients in fifteen separate transplant units in the Los Angeles–Bakersfield–San Diego region of southern California. Tulman remembered that in a recent conversation

Barbara Nuesse had mentioned a patient in one of her hospitals who sounded right for Jacesohn's liver.

"Barbara, I may have a liver for that girl you were telling me about last week."

"Julie Bornn?" answered Nuesse.

"Yes, that's the one," said Tulman. "Is she still alive?"

"Barely," Nuesse answered. There was a note of sadness in her voice.

"How old is she, Barb?" asked Tulman.

"Fourteen."

"And how much does she weigh?"

"Last Thursday she weighed one hundred fourteen pounds, but she's lost a lot of weight. She's a big girl for her age."

"She could be just right," said Tulman. The coordinator for the UCSF transplant unit then read the same medical data to Nuesse that she had given to Marguerite Brown.

"Sounds perfect," said Nuesse. "I'll notify Brems and reserve a Lear." John Brems is a surgeon at UCLA, the major liver transplant center in the region.

Nuesse had four Lear jets at her disposal, ready to fly anywhere in the country to fetch a liver for Julie Bornn. The Lear pilots would charge between $1,000 and $1,500 an hour, and Julie Bornn's parents would have to pay for it. But that seemed a minor item on what would eventually be a $300,000 medical bill.

Lisa Tulman's last call was to Shane De Vine at the Neuroskeletal Transplantation Laboratory in San Jose, California. De Vine's bank collects bone, skin, middle ears, cartilage, and corneas. It stores and distributes them for "a modest procurement and processing fee" to surgeons and hospitals, which use them for reconstructive and perioperative surgeries (small surgical procedures that take place during larger operations). Bone and tissue banking is a subspecialty within organ transplanting, a field about which many organ transplanters are deeply concerned. It's a completely unregulated, profitable industry, that has attracted a number of free-enterprise visionaries and profiteers. "If there is to be a transplant scandal," says De Vine, who sees himself as a reformer in his own trade, "it will be in tissue banking."

De Vine was out, so Tulman left a message. "Would you please tell him that there may be a donor at S.F. General. He hasn't been declared yet. I'll call back when I know details."

Tulman could now return to her own selection process. After a quick scan of her computer-generated list of medically acceptable patients, Tulman found several people who could use one of Jacesohn's kidneys. She paged Dr. Feduska, the surgeon on call.

Nicholas Feduska, an affable Pennsylvania-raised Ukrainian-American, was grabbing a quick lunch, sitting where he always did, next to the phone in the staff cafeteria. When his beeper sounded, he checked the number on its screen, leaned back with a mouthful of salad, and dialed Tulman's number. "Lisa, what's up."

"Nick, there may be a donor at S.F. General," said Tulman.

"What's his status?" Feduska listened carefully to the data Tulman read him on Walden. At least six patients came to mind as possible recipients while he listened to Jacesohn's blood type and other vital statistics. "I'll be right up." He left his lunch on the table and ran to the elevator.

Meanwhile, at San Francisco General, Jacesohn Walden's condition had worsened. But he still had not been declared dead, nor had his family even discussed the subject of organ donation.

Sometime later that day, Jonathan Hodes became convinced that Jacesohn wasn't going to make it. Again he contacted Carol Fink. Together they agreed that it would be appropriate to raise with the Waldens the subject of organ donation.

While surveys of neurosurgeons and neurologists indicate that they overwhelmingly support the concept of brain death, many are still not completely comfortable declaring it. Even less are they comfortable asking for organs. To some degree it is a signal of failure for neurosurgeons to declare brain death. It is, after all, *their* organ and *their* effort to save it that have failed. Why should they feel comfortable passing their patient to transplant surgeons? Similar polls also indicate that there remains in the neurological community a latent fear of legal action, despite the passage of "brain death" laws in forty-two states and solid case law in the others that essentially makes "irreversible" function of the brain a diagnostic sign of death.

At 6:00 P.M. on Sunday, March 1, Dr. Hodes approached Sam Walden and told him for the first time that his son Jacesohn might die. Though Hodes also suggested, as sensitively as he could, that he and Virginia might want to discuss the possibility of organ donation, it would, be up to Carol Fink to make the formal request.

This work was not something Fink prepared for when she became a psychiatric nurse twenty-three years before. Her role as a "transplant liaison" began, she says, about eight years ago, when a transplant coordinator from the University of California, San Francisco, Medical Center began coming over to her hospital and talking to the families of brain-injured patients. "Well, I'm quite territorial about my waiting room," says Fink, "and I resented someone coming in from outside talking to my patients about donating organs." After a brief altercation with the UCSF coordinator, she and Fink developed an agreement whereby Fink would notify her when a potential donor was in her ward, but only Fink could talk with the family.

Today, the process of converting nurses to agents of organ procurement is formalized—"medical marketing," one proponent calls it. In the San Francisco Bay Area medical marketing of organ donation takes the form of a two-day in-service training course designed to convince medical professionals in and around intensive care units to be on the lookout for potential organ donors. Although there would seem to be some inherent conflict between caring for the loved ones of a dying patient and arranging for the removal of his or her organs, Carol Fink has taken the course and appears to accept the medical profession's two-part role as another of the many paradoxes facing modern healthcare.

At about 10:40 A.M. on March 2, 1987, Fink began the long,

familiar walk to the room where relatives wait for word. Though she was specially trained for this moment and had faced hundreds of loved ones before, it was still hard to approach the family of a dying patient and ask for organs—particularly those of the son of the Waldens, a family she came to like and admire so much in a short period of time. It was always hardest when the deceased was a child.

Studies of this unusually tense moment in human interaction have shown that women get considerably better results requesting donation than men. This discovery was probably a tremendous relief to neurosurgeons, most of whom are men and few of whom are comfortable asking for organs. The same surveys have found that requesters of either gender who are not philosophically enthusiastic about organ procurement and transplantation have returns approaching zero.

When Carol Fink reached the end of the hall, she entered the room with confidence. Sam Walden stood up. Virginia clasped her hands. Fink pulled up a chair and asked Sam to sit down. "I have been talking with Dr. Hodes," she said slowly. The care and kindness that showed in her eyes came naturally to her. "He says it doesn't look so good. We don't think Jacesohn's going to make it." She paused until it seemed appropriate to add, "You should consider whether or not you wish to donate his organs." Although required by state law to say that, she did so with a sincerity that came straight from the heart. Fink was raised in an orthodox Jewish family that believed removal of organs could spoil, if not prevent, a resurrection, but she has nevertheless become completely supportive of organ donation and transplantation.

"At first, Virginia Walden did not seem comfortable with the idea," Fink recalls. "But they had time to think about it. Sam was more positive, although he was not too enthusiastic about donating his son's heart. The next day they came back and said they would donate all organs. 'I hope something good will come of this difficult life,' Virginia told me."

By 10:00 P.M. on Sunday, March 1, Jacesohn's EEG had been flat for twenty-two hours, his pupils remained dilated and fixed, and there was still no response to painful stimuli. Another test was tried. A solution of ice water was poured in his ear. There was no reflex reaction. All but one of the criteria on the hospital's strict brain-death list had been checked "negative." There was one last test to perform.

When the edema was found in Jacesohn's brain, he was administered doses of phenobarbital large enough to put him into a barbiturate coma. Since a barbiturate coma has many of the same symptoms as brain death, a special "isotope" scan had to be taken of his head after a radioactive dye had been injected into the artery that carries blood to the brain. The scan showed no blood flow to any part of Jacesohn's brain, a certain sign of "total and irreversible cessation of brain function"—the condition legislated by the state of California as a legal definition of death.

At 11:05 on the night of March 2, Jacesohn Walden was pronounced dead by Jon Hodes. As he signed his patient's death certificate, Hodes instructed the nurses on duty to leave Jacesohn on the respirator that helped oxygen-rich blood circulate throughout his body. Fifteen minutes later, at 11:20, Dr. Boyd Stephens, coroner of San Francisco County, received a call from the hospital requesting permission to harvest organs. Permission was granted. Within forty-eight hours the mortal remains of Jacesohn Walden—his heart, kidneys, liver, corneas, boncs, ligaments, and cartilage—would be pumping, filtering, metabolizing, and otherwise performing their appointed functions in the bodies of more than three dozen living Americans, from upstate New York to Arizona.

CHAPTER 2

THE HARVEST

*The dead body has unlimited use for the imaginative
living.*

ROBERT VEATCH, PH.D.,
Georgetown University

*Closure: Each family member must be permitted private
time with the love one and should be encouraged to say
everything that he/she has always wanted to tell the
patient. Individual personal relationships with the donor
must be completed by each family member so that it is
possible to again assume the threads of his/her own life.
After saying good-bye, most families will wish to leave
the hospital before the transplant team arrives to take the
donor to surgery.*

PHYLLIS WEBER,
Chief Transplant Coordinator,
Northern California Transplant Bank

4:15 P.M., Sunday, March 1, 1987.   After signing the formal
release that allows the hospital to remove Jacesohn's organs and
tissues, Sam and Virginia Walden are invited to return to the
intensive care unit (ICU) one last time—to say good-bye.

The Waldens pause and say they want to think about it for

a while. They have been told that though Jacesohn has been declared dead, they will find him as they had last seen him: his chest still rising and falling rhythmically, his heart beating strongly, his skin still pink and warm to the touch. He won't seem dead.

Doctors and ICU nurses who wholeheartedly accept the concept of brain death (and most do) still comment on the strange sensation that a respirated cadaver presents. The terms they often use to describe patients in Jacesohn's condition—"neomorts" or "biomorts"—suggest a being neither living nor dead, perhaps somewhere in between. It is a confusion that is exacerbated for many ICU staffers by a common occurrence in their wards. When a brain-dead organ donor goes into cardiac arrest, an alarm goes off, and an elaborate protocol of rescue begins. To a bystander it all looks like a desperate attempt to save the patient's life. It is not. It is done only to preserve organs. Ironically, it can take place in the same section of a hospital where a conscious living patient will lie in a bed over which hangs a sign saying DO NOT RECUSITATE.

Early Monday Morning, March 2.   Virginia Walden decides not to return. But at about 10:00 A.M. Sam Walden leaves work to visit the bedside of his son. He returns several times throughout the day.

In the early evening, while he stands alone by Jacesohn's bed for the last time, Nick Feduska scrubs for surgery in a room nearby. Feduska is there for the kidneys, though it will be many hours before he leaves the hospital. He will wait and watch while surgical teams from Stanford and Los Angeles, now en route to San Francisco, arrive to take the heart and liver first. He will assist them and learn more about "sequencing," the order in which organs are removed, and perhaps discuss the new "rapid technique" developed at the University of Pittsburgh—both vital topics in the world of multiple-organ retrieval.

Now that Jacesohn is on donor protocol and all the right fluids are being infused at all the right volumes, the pace of events at his bedside has temporarily slowed. His vital signs—pulse, blood pressure, temperature, and urine output—are occasionally checked by a nurse. A blood sample or two is removed, one to check the nitrogen level, another to be certain the donor isn't carrying any viruses (hepatitis and AIDS being the most worrisome) that could be transmitted to a recipient or a surgeon.

High over the coastal mountains of California, a Lear jet carries the UCLA liver procurement team. There are three aboard besides the pilots: surgical resident John Brems, the lead surgeon on this trip; another resident; and a nurse. Like the other teams, they come with their own instruments, chemicals, and ice chest to carry their organ home. The flight gives the doctors an hour to rest and prepare for a long, sleepless night. Some surgeons believe that the removal of a donor's organ is as vital to success as the implant operation. But the run for a donor organ is a stressful assignment, one tinged with sadness. Therefore it's often the first to be passed on to a transplant unit's residents. Brems, thirty-three, leans back in his seat and watches the sun set over the Pacific.

Brems has met Feduska at conventions and read most of his many papers on immunosuppression and donor-specific transfusions. But this is the first time they will operate together.

As Brems's jet descends into San Francisco, Marguerite Brown discusses last-minute details with the Stanford cardiac team that is "redballing" north on Highway 101 in a Stanford ambulance. She is anxious to know whether all preparations for the recipient operation are under way at Stanford. Her team has performed as many heart transplants as any in the world, but Brown knows that a single forgotten detail on the long checklist of transplant preparations can have tragic consequences. She is, according to many of her peers, "a pro."

7:45 P.M. Sam Walden leaves the hospital. Carol Fink watches him walk slowly down the long hallway for the last time. She is especially sad at that moment because in their intense five days together, she has grown to like the Waldens more than most families she has worked with.

BIOMORT

9:03 P.M. To an unschooled bystander in a hallway of San Francisco General Hospital, Jacesohn Walden, wheeled by on a gurney, seems no different than a regular patient headed for surgery. Orderlies slide him off the gurney onto the operating table with all the care afforded the living. His vital signs are stable.

A cardiopulmonary machine is wheeled into the operating room. It will take over the essential life-imitating functions. After the heart is removed, blood will be recirculated back into Jacesohn's body, just as it would be were he there for open-heart surgery. In his case, the purpose is to keep liver and kidneys supplied with blood until shortly before they are removed.

9:21 P.M. Jacesohn's slight, muscular young body is carefully shaved and sterilized. His vital signs are checked again while heart monitors are placed on his chest and arms. The anesthesiologist, consulting the checklist on his clipboard, performs his preoperative tasks step by step.

Anesthesia seems perfunctory in a way. Biomorts have shown absolutely no evidence of experiencing pain. But the anesthetic function is not to suppress pain. It is to stabilize blood gases and send a generous supply of oxygen to vital organs. When the organs are removed, anesthesia will cease.

Before the operation begins, as with all major thoracic or abdominal surgeries, Jacesohn is draped in a long surgical blue sheet that is carefully opened and clamped to reveal only the operative field. Once all the tubes, needles, and sensors that will breathe, feed, and monitor Jacesohn are in place, a sterile cloth barrier is placed over his head. No procurement surgeon will ever see his face.

When the scrub nurses and anesthesiologist have finished their preparatory work, the heart team is summoned. Without ceremony, Dr. Philip Oyer from Stanford steps to the table and asks for a scalpel. He makes a long incision from the neck all the way down to the pubis, then another across the midsection from flank to flank, completely exposing the viscera. A surgical saw divides the sternum, which is splayed open with a large mechanical device nicknamed "the iron intern." A strong young heart is revealed, beating a rhythmic sixty-two times a minute according to the top indicator on a bank of screens and charts that monitor vital signs. Beneath the heart is the smooth pink surface of a healthy liver. It could be after midnight before the kidneys are seen. By the following evening these organs will be in the bodies of four living people.

Cannulas (plastic tubes) are placed in the aorta and vena cava (the main arteries and veins running to and from the heart) and connected to the heart-lung machine. The next procedure seems quick and remarkably simple. A cold saline solution is poured over the heart, the aorta is clamped, the ventricles (lower chambers of the heart) are infused with a potassium-rich solution that suddenly stops the heartbeat and begins the preservation process. A few snips and the "seat of life," grayish pink and limp, is cradled in cautious hands and passed from surgeon to nurse, who immerses it in another cold solution that was prepared moments before in a large sterile basin. The last drops of Jacesohn's blood are washed away. His heart is dropped into a plastic jar filled with a clear white electrolyte compound that mimics the functions of intercellular chemicals in the body.

ISCHEMIC TIME

The longer a heart or any other organ can be preserved, the farther it can be transported. The longer surgeons can wait before implanting an organ, the better the chances of finding a well-matched recipient and having him or her prepared for transplant. Researchers at most larger transplant centers are still working to develop optimal preservation technologies for human organs. They experiment only with animal organs, of course. Hearts, livers, kidneys, and pancreases are removed from dogs, cats, pigs, and monkeys with hopes that whatever ischemic (preservation) times can be obtained will approximate those of their human counterparts. One by one they are placed in some new solution or device with hopes of breaking an existing preservation record for a particular organ: heart, eight hours; liver, six hours; kidneys, maybe seventy-two hours.

The key to successful organ preservation, transplanters now believe, is "core-cooling"—rapid infusion with a chilled solution of carefully blended, high-electrolyte composition into the blood-delivery system of the organ. In some cases surgeons will make the infusion as soon as the organ is removed, in others they will cannulate (i.e., insert a plastic tube inside) the vessels leading to the organ and perfuse it before it is even removed. Either way, the objective is to replace the donor's blood and lower the organ temperature as fast as possible.

All sorts of inventions and experiments have been attempted to lengthen ischemic time. A machine under development at the University of Minnesota has preserved kidneys for ninety-six hours. "And we are pushing the envelope beyond that now," says John Heil, Minnesota's perfusion technician and animal lab supervisor. Minnesota now routinely places all its cadaver kidneys on its machine. However, many transplant teams in the U.S. and most in Europe still simply drop them into a plastic bag filled with ice-cold Collins solution (a mixture of potassium phosphate, potassium chloride, and sodium bicarbonate).

"There is no evidence that machines preserve kidneys better or longer than cold solution," says veteran French kidney transplanter René Küss. John Heil says that may be true and even admits that his machines can, and occasionally do, damage kidneys. He still sees the future in machines. "We have reached the max—about seventy-two hours—with cold solution alone. We know we can only go beyond that with [machine-aided] perfusion."

Similar devices have been tested for livers and hearts. But, as with kidney preservation machines, many surgeons have found them to be of little value. Most bizarre of all devices is the "heart-lung box" developed by Drs. Robert Hardesty and Bartley Griffith at the University of Pittsburgh. Lungs remain the most frustrating preservation challenge in transplanting. Heart-lung donors who do not die very close to a transplant center are often flown—brain dead and intact, attached to a cumbersome respirator—to wherever the transplant will be performed. To avoid this expensive and time-consuming procedure, Hardesty and Griffith developed "the box," as it is familiarly known at Pittsburgh. The box is an elaborate device for transporting the supersensitive heart-lung combination long distances.

The theory behind the box is that a heart-lung transplant will be much more successful if fluids are kept flowing, at a normal rate and pressure, through the complex maze of delicate vessels that fill a lung. The pump in the box that moves the cold solution through the vascular system of the lungs is the heart itself, which is kept beating by a complex, electronically controlled mechanism attached to the box. The University of Pittsburgh's public relations department once promoted the box as a great medical advance.

"It doesn't work," says Marguerite Brown, transplant coordinator at Stanford University Hospital, who accompanied the heart team to San Francisco. "They've abandoned it and gone back to the 'Stanford method' [packing the heart and lungs together in a common ice chest]. Of course, they don't call it that," adds Brown, chuckling.

Technological rivalry among transplant units is endemic, as surgical rivalry has been for decades. The patents on a piece of machinery that works could mean millions of dollars to a university or hospital. Pittsburgh chief of transplant surgery Tom

Starzl agrees that there are still some wrinkles to be ironed out of the box. In the meantime, he calls it "a temporary expedient." Tom Chakurda, former spokesman for Pitt, admitted shortly before leaving the university that they never use it anymore.

The best hope for preserving solid organs appears to remain in the chemistry of preservation fluids rather than in devices or machines. At an International Transplant Forum held in September of 1987, Dr. Folkert Belzer of the University of Wisconsin announced that he and his research staff had developed a new ten-ingredient solution that could preserve animal livers for twenty-four hours. If it works on human livers, which can now be kept away from a blood supply for only about six hours, it will advance liver transplantation enormously by allowing donor organs to be transported much farther than they are today and still leave time for tissue typing, which, research has shown, improves the long-term survival rates of all transplanted organs.

Maximizing "cold ischemic time" will always be a major goal of transplanters. If cryogenic researchers ever find a way to deep-freeze and permanently store viable solid organs or biomorts, "the field of transplantation would be absolutely revolutionized overnight," predicts Pittsburgh's Tom Starzl. "With good preservation techniques, worldwide sharing programs could be put into effect."

SECOND THOUGHTS

10:40 P.M.   The tone in Operating Room 6 is decidedly upbeat. None of the surgeons and nurses that bustle around Jacesohn Walden, biomort, ever knew him when he was alive. They didn't treat his wounds or struggle to save his life; nor did they ever meet Sam or Virginia Walden. Jacesohn's purpose now, and theirs, is to save living patients who wait in other cities for his parts.

This is not to suggest that organ harvests are joyous events.

Even veteran transplanters have their moments. "There is an instant, when I am leaving the operating room and look back at that lifeless body on the table, that I am uncomfortable," admits Rob Gordon, a surgeon at the University of Pittsburgh. "But then I look down and see the ice chest and remind myself that what I am carrying will save the life of another."

Marguerite Brown, too, has had her moments. She describes an incident in Los Angeles when, because the team was short one member, she was asked to assist in a multiple-organ retrieval. "It was a young girl, eleven or twelve. Of course, during the operation you are not aware of such details, because all you can see is an open body. Everything else is covered with surgical cloth. But at one moment near the end of the operation, a little blond pigtale appeared from under the blue cloth." Brown, who is blond herself, recalls being "overcome with sadness. I try to stay out of the OR as much as possible now."

10:45 P.M.   While Jacesohn's heart is packed in ice and lowered gently into a red and white picnic cooler, Marguerite Brown is on the phone to Dr. Norman Shumway in Palo Alto. "We'll be moving in less than ten minutes. It's a great-looking heart," Brown tells her boss. Most people in the field say he's the best heart transplanter in the world.

10:50 P.M.   The Stanford heart team packs its instruments and prepares to leave for Palo Alto, where a recipient has been selected and is being anesthetized. The UCLA liver team, scrubbed and gloved, moves over the table. "Looks healthy," says John Brems, gently squeezing Jacesohn's liver.

Brems is a recent arrival to transplanting. He works with a team of five surgeons formed three and a half years earlier by Dr. Ron Busuttil. Brems, a native of Iowa, chose liver transplanting from a host of choices. The year he did so, 1984, only two people applied for the residency he filled at UCLA. "This year," says Brems, "there are more than twenty. Transplanting is hot. It is by far the most-sought-after surgical specialty in American medical schools today."

Removing and transplanting livers is considerably more complex than the same procedures performed on hearts. Not only are there more veins and arteries to sever and tie off, but they are smaller and more fragile. The liver is also such a prodigious container and processor of blood that its removal causes serious blood pressure imbalances throughout the entire body. And there are the gallbladder and biliary tracts to contend with. Furthermore, the liver is attached to the back of the abdominal cavity by a series of sensitive membranes. A slight error in their severance can cause serious bleeding. A surgeon must often work blind, under the liver, taking great care not to damage the organ while severing its frail attachments.

So the liver team will take much longer than the heart team, carefully tying off each vein and artery as the removal slowly proceeds. Following a method developed at the University of Pittsburgh and adopted almost overnight worldwide, the superior mesenteric vein is cannulated so that a cold preservation fluid can be pumped into all remaining organs as soon as the heart-lung machine is removed. The liver and kidneys will thus be "core-cooled" until they are removed from the donor.

11:40 P.M. "Liver's out," says Brems as he turns to hand the now steel gray organ to an assistant. Like the heart when it is taken out, the liver is immediately washed and flushed with a solution that removes the last of Jacesohn's blood from inside and outside the organ. Once cleaned, it is packed in a picnic cooler, this one blue, and chilled to 0°.

Tossing their rubber gloves, masks, and blood-soaked robes into a sterile bin, Brems and his team grab the cooler and run through the halls of the hospital. The elevator is currently on the eighth floor. They're waiting on the third. The elevator is very slow. They take to the stairs.

Behind the hospital an ambulance waits to rush them to the

airport at full siren. The Lear is revved up and waiting on the end of the tarmac. The small plane gets immediate clearance, makes its characteristic short takeoff, and climbs steeply to cruising altitude for a fifty-five-minute flight south to Van Nuys, a small town east of Los Angeles. At first, members of the team try to grab a few moments' sleep, but adrenaline keeps them awake. Half a dozen jokes and a Pepsi later, they are on the ground.

At Van Nuys, a helicopter waits to take Brems and the liver to a rooftop heliport at UCLA Medical Center, where a carefully screened and selected recipient is open on the operating table. Brems, who has already been awake for eighteen hours, will sew. It's not uncommon for liver transplant surgeons to go thirty-six hours without sleep, especially when a surgeon both procures and implants a given organ.

PANCREASES

Had Jacesohn's pancreas been removed, it would have been taken before the liver. But the removal of the pancreas can damage the liver, making it useless for transplantation. Naturally, liver transplanters get upset about this. Why "knowingly sacrifice a liver" that could save a patient's life, asks Pittsburgh's liver impresario, Tom Starzl, "in order to provide a luxury for a pancreas recipient who has the option of insulin therapy?" Starzl angrily points to unidentified parts of the country where "two-, three-, four-year-old donors are used to obtain pancreases to put into adult diabetics; something which, at its core, I believe is profoundly unethical, and it cannot go on."

Dr. Nancy Ascher, head of the newly formed liver transplant unit at UCSF, says that when she was at the University of Minnesota, where pancreases are frequently harvested from cadavers for transplantation, her team developed a successful technique for retrieving both pancreas and liver. "There are a few cases where anatomical difficulties will make it impossible to take both organs," she says, "but eighty percent of the time we were able to recover both successfully."

Since there is not much pancreas transplantation in the San Francisco Bay Area, this was not even an issue in the Walden case. Coincidentally, kidney transplant surgeon Julie Melzer of UCSF expressed her intention to begin transplanting the pancreas in January 1988, about the same time that Nancy Ascher arrived from Minneapolis to open the liver unit there. So far, there have been no conflicts of interest between them.

12:05 A.M. March 3, 1987. Nick Feduska steps to the table to remove Jacesohn's kidneys. The crowd in Operating Room 6 has thinned considerably and an atmosphere of exhaustion prevails. Feduska, however, seems tireless. He runs on adrenaline, he says, and recounts Memorial Day weekend in 1984, when he stayed up for forty-eight hours retrieving kidneys from Santa Rosa to Fresno and performing four separate transplants.

A constant stream of friendly chatter and jokes (none at the expense of the deceased) flow from under Feduska's mask. He keeps the team awake and alert for the last hour of a long night.

Nick Feduska is part of the new breed, a "second-generation" transplanter. While he trained, he watched the laity react to the practices and policies of his mentors. Public reaction, he observed, was not always positive. So Feduska is more conservative than his elders. He is careful about the semantics of what he says. He *never*, for example, uses the word "harvest" in his papers or conversations. He prefers "recovery" and encourages his peers at UCSF to use it in their communications. "At the University of Pittsburgh, where I did my residence, surgeons were pretty insensitive about terms and things they would discuss around patients and family," Feduska recalls. "I'm not a complete believer in holistic medicine, but I do believe that the attitude of a physician is important to the health of his patients."

Things have changed little in Pittsburgh since Feduska left.

Thomas Starzl, the feisty and controversial chief of transplant surgery, still uses the word "harvest" in his papers and conversations, even after his former transplant coordinator, Donald Denny, switched to "retrieve" one day in 1983 when an irate physician (not a transplanter) shrieked at him that no one was going to "harvest" one of his patients "as though he were a cash crop." Denny attempted to convert Starzl and his peers to more prudent usage, but to no avail. Words like "harvest" and "procurement" are still in common use in medical literature and throughout the transplant community.

THE LAST RITE OF HARVEST

Kidneys are fairly easy to remove. In some centers the operation is done by an intern, even a paramedic. But Feduska has learned from sad experience that little things can go wrong—trauma to an artery, an improper cut on the ureter, or abrasion of the delicate intima (inner lining) of the renal vein. So he insists that all kidneys coming to his center be removed by surgeons, and when at all possible, he himself prefers to be the surgeon.

He enjoys this part of his work, particularly the teamwork. "It has always amazed me," he says, "that three separate teams which may never have worked together before can come into a small hospital that may never have done a donor before, and get along so well."

12:10 A.M. With the heart and liver gone, there is more room to work. The peritoneum is divided and the bowel moved to one side, exposing two healthy kidneys. Vessels leading to and from the kidneys are isolated, cannulated, and perfused with preserving solutions. The kidneys are removed en bloc (as a unit), still attached to their main vessels. They are lowered gently into a pan of cold solution, washed clean of blood, and attached to a perfusion machine similar to the one developed at Minnesota.

The machine, a clear-plastic covered box standing about eighteen inches high, will gently pump a cool preservative through both kidneys until they are transplanted, sometime within the next forty-eight hours.

12:55 A.M. The major solid organs are out and en route to new owners in Los Angeles, Palo Alto, and San Francisco. Next come the corneas, which Feduska stays to remove as a favor to the eye bank. When he is finished, a three-member team from the Neuroskeletal Transplantation Laboratory arrive to remove some bone and connective tissue that will be processed, sterilized at their facilities in San Jose, and distributed to surgeons, hospitals, and medical centers. Most of the tissues will be used for reconstructive surgeries.

The tissue-harvesting team operate at a more relaxed pace than the organ harvesters, who bear the constant pressure of short ischemic times and dying patients at the other end. Bone and most nonvascular tissues can be safely removed from a cadaver by trained technicians any time within the first twenty-four hours after death—and it needn't be from a beating-heart cadaver. Almost any healthy human can be a tissue donor, no matter how he or she dies. But most people who donate their solid organs also become tissue donors. When the request is made for organs, tissues are generally listed in the consent form.

Before they leave San Francisco, the NTL team carefully inserts wooden dowels about the width of broomsticks where Jacesohn's long bones had been. They then close their incisions with sutures just as they would following a regular operation. It is their policy, as it is with most tissue bankers, to leave the deceased appearing completely intact, in case the family decides to have an open-coffin funeral.

The entire harvest lasts just over eight hours; about average. It can take considerably longer with less skilled personnel or if complications develop. And it can be done a lot quicker if need be. The October 1987 edition of *Surgery, Gynecology and Ob-*

stetrics contains an article describing a "rapid technique for multiple organ harvesting which allows removal of all major organs within 30 to 60 minutes after beginning the donor operation." (Notice the use of "harvest" in a contemporary medical paper.) Developed by Thomas Starzl and his team at the University of Pittsburgh, the rapid technique has been widely acclaimed and is now in common use at several centers. The method involves cooling "the organs by infusion of cold solutions in situ [while they are still in the patient] with subsequent rapid dissection in a bloodless field."

John Brems has tried the technique, and says it works well, but prefers the slower method used with Jacesohn Walden. "If the donor is unstable and we stand a chance of loosing the organs by waiting, the rapid method is great. But if he's stable and we can carefully dissect the vessels, it's easier to work at the other end. Also, as soon as you clamp the aorta, the ischemic time begins. Well, you have to clamp the aorta right away with the rapid technique, so ironically you have less time left at the end of the procedure than with the longer technique, where the liver has blood flow almost up to the moment it is removed."

1:25 A.M. Jacesohn Walden's body, now almost twenty pounds lighter than when he died, is stitched up and washed. A nurse calls the funeral home, and heads to her own home for a well-earned night of sleep.

CHAPTER 3

THE WAITING

Shall organs go to the sickest, or to the ones with most promise of recovery; on a first come first served basis; to the most valuable patient (based on wealth, education position, what?); to the one with the most dependents; to women and children first; to those who can pay?

Or *should lots be cast?*

JAMES FLETCHER,
American ethicist

As the system has evolved, each American transplant patient now waits on at least one list, in at least one major transplant center somewhere in the country. If centers are complying with regulations, they will also be registered with the United Network for Organ Sharing. On the day of Jacesohn's death, there were 677 patients on Dr. Nick Feduska's kidney list in San Francisco. Twenty-six waited for hearts at Stanford and thirty-one were on the UCLA hospital liver list.

While Jonathan Hodes and his neurological staff at San Francisco General Hospital were still making valorous attempts to save Jacesohn's life, separate selection processes for each of his organs were well under way at all three of the hospitals selected to receive organs. No two transplant units make their final selections in quite the same way. At UCLA the choice is made by committee, at UCSF and Stanford, by the attending surgeon. But

27

whatever the selection process, the result would be the same in the Jacesohn Walden case: only six fewer people would be left on waiting lists.

On March 2, 1987, Nick Feduska still defended his right to transplant any organ he "recovers" to anyone his choses. To him that didn't mean he "owns" the kidney. Instead, he said, "I am holding it in trust."

The morning after he removed Jacesohn Walden's kidney, Feduska came to work early. Lisa Tulman, UCSF's chief transplant coordinator, had already been at work for more than half an hour gathering the charts on all patients who could conceivably accept Jacesohn's kidneys. Feduska took off a tweed jacket and slipped into his long white coat. The first arm through a sleeve reached for the phone. He punched two numbers. "Lisa, you ready? . . . Okay, come on in."

Before Feduska arrived, Tulman had entered Jacesohn's blood and tissue type into her computer and received a printout of eleven names (from the list of 677) potential recipients. It was the complete charts on those eleven patients that she brought to the meeting; the stack was almost two feet high. One by one, Feduska and Tulman leafed through the thick file on each patient.

"Does she still live in Humboldt?" Feduska asked of one.

"Yes," answered Tulman.

"Well, she's pretty far away. I'm not sure she can make it down here in time. Let's pass on her for now. Besides, she seems to be doing well on dialysis."

Proximity to the hospital, Feduska explained, is a factor at most centers. While it does discriminate against people in outlying areas, there is justification for it when an organ has already been ischemic (out of the body) for a few hours, as was the case with Jacesohn's kidneys. The successful ongoing dialysis of the Humboldt patient simply assured Feduska and Tulman that it wouldn't hurt her medically to wait for another kidney.

"Now, as I recall, we had some trouble with this guy's compliance," said Feduska, holding up the next file.

"That's right," said Tulman, "he wouldn't take his medicine."
"Now, that becomes a very important consideration after a transplant," Feduska explained. "If this patient doesn't follow a strict regimen of immunosuppression, he will lose his graft and we will have wasted a kidney." He turned to Tulman. "Lisa, please call his physician and ask if his compliance has improved. If it hasn't, you might mention that he was passed over for that reason.

"Here's a patient who has only been on the list for three weeks. She's in fair health and doing well on dialysis. Let's have her wait for a while."

The next file was for a man who lived in a tough, high-crime neighborhood in nearby Oakland. "Now, I would not exclude this patient because of his address," said Feduska. "That would be 'red-lining.' But the last time I saw him he had fresh needle tracks on his upper arm—and they were not from dialysis. He admits that he was once a heroin addict, and I am afraid he might have gone back to it. We just can't risk transplanting him until we are sure about his habit."

The issue of whether or not an organ disease is self-induced is a big one in transplanting. "Why should we waste a liver on a man who destroyed the one God gave him with alcohol?" one surgeon might ask. "Because our oath as physicians mandates us to treat the sick no matter what the etiology of his disease," another could answer.

"Now, here's a good candidate," said Tulman, handing Feduska the next file. "He has been waiting for almost eighteen months, is extremely compliant, and lives in the city. He came in for a visit last week and looked strong.

"This guy has four children and is only able to work part time because dialysis kind of sets him back for a few hours after every session. I think he will do very well with a new kidney and might be able to get back to full-time work. Put him on the short list." Tulman set his file on the corner of the desk.

"Here's Olivia Hernandez again. Remember, she rejected

her sister's kidney and is back on dialysis. Her PRA [panel re-active antibody] has dropped ten points since we last saw her and she can be here in four hours.'' Feduska nodded and the Her-nandez file, too, was placed on the corner of the desk.

By the end of the meeting, which lasted about an hour, eight of the eleven medically qualified candidates were placed back on the waiting list. There were three "winners" and two kidneys. There was one extra because Tulman has learned from experience that one of the three will be unable to make it in time for a transplant. She would call them in the order Feduska determined.

THE LIST

At the moment of Jacesohn's death, there were close to 20,000 Americans waiting for his parts. His most vital organs—heart and liver—would save only two of them, leaving thousands to wait on in desperation. His kidneys and corneas would be shared among four recipients.

Only two or three thousand of the 20,000 candidates were on the verge of death. Perhaps a thousand others, with heart and liver diseases, although not yet classified "terminal," had been given a few months, maybe a year or two, to live. Another 8,000 (those who awaited kidneys) were being maintained on dialysis. Among them were patients with slow, degenerative organ dis-eases brought on by diabetes, many of whom had been waiting for years.

More than half of the heart and liver patients who were on waiting lists when Jacesohn died were never transplanted and died during the year that followed. To those who survived and took the time to study available statistics, the odds became clear and the despair for some became unbearable. In July of 1987 a sixty-year-old Long Island jewler named Joseph Rizzo confessed to *New York* magazine that he had "prayed for an accident to kill a healthy young person his size and blood type so that he might have a new heart.''

THE NETWORK

Two separate selection processes take place for each donated organ. First, a transplant center must be chosen. That will be done by a regional organ procurement agency, sometimes working in concert with a national computer center that is attempting to register all candidates for transplantation. Once a center is found, a recipient must be selected from its waiting list. That is done either by a chief surgeon or by a committee of surgeons and staff at the hospital.

Jacesohn's organs could conceivably have ended up anywhere in the world. The fact that they remained in the United States and were all transplanted in California reflects a distribution system that has evolved over the past thirty years. It wasn't always as fair and democratic as it is today.

Here is how Thomas Starzl, veteran transplanter and possibly the best-known surgeon in the field, describes the organ procurement system of earlier days: "With the explosion of demand [in the early 1970s] came great 'star wars' fought out worldwide over these so-called 'franchises.' What began as a crusade became a business in which medical titans found themselves in gladiatorial conflict."

What Starzl witnessed, and for a time accepted, was a chaotic morass of organizations, agencies, hospitals, societies, entrepreneurs, and surgeons, all competing for cadaver organs. They played a sort of feudal board game where the aristocracy of transplantation (surgeons) sent minions (transplant coordinators, organ procurement specialists, and "consultants") out to do battle over scarce "franchises." The mission of transplantation's lieutenants was to bring back as many organs as possible. It didn't really matter how or how many. The more organs a transplant center could procure, the more patients would seek its services.

The system became rife with favoritism (wherein the famous and telegenic were selected over the anonymous and the poor), veiled threats (pressuring organ procurement agencies to provide organs by threatening to withhold endorsements for licensing), and the cutting of deals (paying a "finder's fee" to trauma unit staffers who called a transplant unit when a trauma patient was close to brain death). Organ procurement took on all the trappings of a Wall Street enterprise—expensive lunches, lavish parties, and insider trading. Aggression was rewarded, not friendly persuasion. Organs went to the best "sales force," and not always to the best centers.

By 1984 organ distribution became so random and inequitable that it began to damage the cause of transplantation. Two congressional committees announced plans to investigate the situation and scheduled hearings. Meanwhile, a quiet but determined reform movement began to emerge within the transplant community itself. Reformers, most of them transplant coordinators and staffers in the 110 organ procurement agencies (OPAs) scattered throughout the country, became determined to combat the entrenched physician-centered apparatus so aptly described by Starzl. OPA workers were naturally the first to see the injustices and dangers of an anarchic "old boy network," but felt powerless to correct it. Many became demoralized and moved on to other fields of healthcare. Others, like Gayle Rogers, stayed to fight.

"We are *still* operating in an old boy network," Rogers lamented in June of 1987, "but things have definitely improved." She works at the St. Paul, Minnesota, Red Cross, which coordinates organ procurement in the five-state area surrounding Minneapolis, the other major transplant center in the U.S. "As a consequence of the old boy approach to organ procurement, places like Pittsburgh still get an inordinate share of organs." Pittsburgh, she says, was dubbed a "black hole" by her peers. By that they simply meant that "a lot of organs went there, but none came out."

PITT

The University of Pittsburgh, where Tom Starzl directs transplanting, became a "black hole" for reasons fortuitous, noble and ignoble. Once Henry Bahnson, the university's chief of surgery, had made a departmental commitment to support a large multiorgan transplant center, Pittsburgh's transplant unit grew fast. The city is located one hour's flying distance from 70% of the American population, making the hospital an ideal site for organ procurement. Add to that a well-funded, aggressive, hospital-based procurement team that was willing to fly thousands of miles at a moment's notice, state-of-the-art laboratories, ongoing research support, teams of surgeons committed to operating at all hours of the night—and you had a transplant center that soon became a net importer of human organs.

Transplant coordinators 2,000 miles from Pittsburgh would come to work in the morning to hear that Starzl's team had done a midnight multiple-organ harvest thirty miles away from their center. While civic pride blossomed in Pittsburgh over a new growth industry, resentment bloomed in Kansas.

Gayle Rogers and her colleagues in organ procurement sought to convince the surgeons and physicians they served that without fairness and equitable distribution of organs, their practice, which had become so dependent on nationwide voluntary donations and on cooperation between hospitals, would eventually collapse. After years of ignoring the advice and admonitions of people like Rogers, and even their own transplant coordinators, surgeons and hospital administrators began to see that the "black hole" system was good for some but ultimately counterproductive to the national transplant effort.

In 1984 the United Network for Organ Sharing (UNOS) was formed in Richmond, Virginia. Reflecting a compromise between surgeons and transplant coordinators, UNOS became the first national organ distribution network in the U.S., modeling itself on countrywide systems that had been operating successfully in Europe for the previous ten years.

In 1986 UNOS was selected by the Reagan administration to receive a million-dollar federal grant to coordinate all organ distribution and enforce fairness. Inspired and encouraged by the National Association of Transplant Coordinators, UNOS was expected to bring an end to the old boy network. In an unexpected and unprecedented move, the American Society of Transplant Surgeons voted to support federally mandated reforms, to be enforced by UNOS, that called for a maximum of one independent organ procurement agency in every region; open sharing of organs within each region; the registration of all transplant patients and donors on a nationwide computer system managed by UNOS; and a final selection of recipients based on a point system reflecting strict medical criteria.

UNOS is now in twenty-four-hour two-way communication with 226 transplant centers and 63 organ procurement agencies across the country. Through computer terminals stationed in each location, the network attempts to coordinate a system redesigned to regulate competition for organs and enhance the fairest possible nationwide distribution of supplies. By the end of February 1988, UNOS had registered almost 14,000 patients, a number that is believed to represent close to 100% of the patients on all waiting lists in the country.

Before the reforms, surgeons argued that if they seemed aggressive it was only because they were acting in the interest of very sick patients. A surgeon would be less willing to acknowledge, perhaps, that pride, economics, and ego also played their parts (and still do) in the selection process. There is money, power, and glory in human organ transplants. Most would add that as bad as the system became, no real scandal ever touched their units—with the possible exception of the Pittsburgh's transplant center.

PITTSBURGH PRESS

In June of 1985 the University of Pittsburgh, by then the largest transplant center in the world, received a near-fatal overdose of public exposure. The entire American transplant community was still reeling from it a year later, and its revelations have since been added to the agenda of ethical issues debated by transplanters the world over.

Widely publicized charges of patient favoritism and financial abuse engendered so much indignation, first in Pittsburgh but ultimately nationwide, that the Justice Department initiated a federal grand jury investigation of the hospital and its practices. By early 1988 the jury was still hearing witnesses and deliberating whether to bring indictments against American transplant surgeons and hospital administrators.

It began with a series of Pulitzer Prize–winning articles in the *Pittsburgh Press* that documented practices later found not to be exclusive to Pittsburgh. Not only did Thomas Starzl's world-class team play favorites in its selection of organ recipients, the *Press* reported, but the favorites were often rich foreigners who were moved past dying Americans and transplanted with organs donated by American families. The foreigners, often Saudis, were then being billed about four times the normal rate for a transplant. One Saudi prince, the paper revealed, after his daughter had received two kidneys from Starzl's team, not only paid the inflated bill but also made a $650,000 donation to the university.

One of the most vexing ethical quandaries facing American transplanters has since become the matter of sharing organs with foreigners. Should organs donated by Americans go only to Americans? Should foreigners be allowed to come here, as they do for other surgical procedures, and participate in our organ procurement network? Or should we only transplant people who bring an organ with them (or a related donor)? Should foreigners be charged the same fee and hospital costs as Americans? Should American organs be shipped overseas? And should exported organs meet the same quality specifications as those transplanted here?

Grand jurists have heard testimony not only that the Saudi princess received a kidney donated by an American who was told it would go to an American, but also that most of the 200 to 250 American cadaver kidneys shipped overseas for transplantation (not into princesses) were unsuitable for use anywhere. These organs were what Tom Starzl labeled, in a follow-up interview with the *Pittsburgh Press*, "crumb kidneys," one of which he even admitted transplanting into the wife of the financial advisor to King Faud of Saudi Arabia. Starzl's Saudi patients were understandably more aghast at this announcment than at the news that they had been grossly overbilled.

The bold admission that the most prestigious American transplant center was dumping inferior kidneys on the rest of the world did little to improve foreign relations for Pittsburgh or the United States. Public indignation went international, and eventually Pittsburgh lost its veteran transplant coordinator, Donald Denny, who left the hospital in disgust in December of 1985.

Largely in response to the nationwide front-page and evening-news coverage that flowed from the Pittsburgh stories, the National Task Force on Organ Transplantation, which was appointed by President Reagan to examine the entire national transplant process, issued a recommendation that a maximum of 10% of transplants at each center should be performed for foreign nationals. The American Society of Transplant Surgeons lowered that recommendation to 5%.

In response to the scandal that rocked the University of Pittsburgh's transplant unit, Tom Starzl completely revised his entire selection system for cadaver kidney recipients, shifting from a surgeon-dominated committee that often reviewed patient selections after the fact (i.e., after the transplant) to a sophisticated, computerized selection system that gives numerical weight to strictly objective medical considerations like waiting time, antigen match, antibody analysis, medical urgency, and logistical practicality. Each of the criteria is applied equally to each patient on the hospital's waiting list. The Pittsburgh point system— detailed in a June 12, 1987, article authored by Starzl in the *Journal of the American Medical Association*—has been widely read and discussed in the transplant community. Ironically, the Pittsburgh system is being emulated around the country by some of Tom Starzl's most vocal critics. It is required by UNOS.

The brilliance of the Pittsburgh system is that it loads all existing selection criteria into a single decision hierarchy that is administered impartially by a computer. No longer can a recipient be selected because he has a nice family, a prestigious position, or an impressive athletic career; or rejected because she was once a prostitute. The only subjective judgment remains the numerical weight placed on criteria. But since whatever weight is finally placed on each criterion remains constant with all patients, the system is much fairer than it was—thanks to public pressure.

Starzl, who said at the time of their publication that the *Pittsburgh Press* articles were unfair and distorted, now attributes his and other reforms in the transplant industry to their publication.

GOLIATHS AND DAVIDS

Today, waiting patients and their families are assured that they will move up the list according to UNOS rules and be selected by medical criteria. But the savvy among them also realize that the UNOS system is still a limited one and that their chances of being selected can be improved with a little creativity and effort.

Transplant consumers are more informed today than than they were before two separate national service organizations were formed on their behalf. One, the Transplant Recipients International Organization, based in Pittsburgh, was founded by a group of former patients from the university's transplant center and provides advise, counseling, and emotional support to transplant patients. The Children's Transplant Association, based in Laurinburg, North Carolina, tends to be more of a reform-minded organization, lobbying Washington, state legislatures, insurance companies, and transplant organizations on behalf of patients and their families.

From both organizations' newsletters, patients and families have learned that, despite the UNOS reforms and enforcement, they still might be chosen in the end by the surgeon or transplant team that harvests the donor organ. Who that surgeon is will depend on a rotating system determined by the Independent Organ Procurement Agency (IOPA) licensed to operate in that region.

If ailing patients waiting for organs study the system closely, they will find that the rotation arrangement in one region may favor the largest center, in another the newest center. Either way, they will be stuck with a tough consumer choice: Should I register at the large center, where I may wait longer but get more professional care, or at the smaller center, where I'll get an organ faster but have less experienced surgeons? Or should I register at both?

Some of Nick Feduska's 680 patients might well ask themselves that question. With the new rotation system in the northern California region, patients could wait months, even years, for a new kidney at UCSF. On the other hand, they could possibly get transplanted much faster at Herrick Memorial hospital across the bay in Oakland, or up the road in Santa Rosa, where the general hospital just opened a new transplant unit. But would they get the postoperative medical attention they need, or the surgical experience of over 3,000 transplants performed at UCSF?

Feduska, who wholeheartedly supports the UNOS reforms, is nonetheless fighting for his patients. He describes a meeting of representatives from all the transplant units in the region, held in November of 1987: "I proposed that we establish a point system to allocate cadaver donor kidneys when they became available. My system would take into account the number of people on waiting lists and the number of transplants a unit had performed over the past twelve months. Well, the other units in the region thought my idea was offensive. They saw it as a classic David-and-Goliath proposal."

And of course they were partly right. The University of California is the Goliath of kidney transplantation—the largest unit in the world, which means, at least in terms of sheer numbers, that it is also the most experienced. And to Feduska, that is a factor worth considering in the allocation of scarce resources.

Even with the certainty of a longer wait, UCSF has more patients on its kidney list than all other hospitals in the region combined. Feduska naturally fears that a rotation system which does not take that into account will force his patients to wait even longer than they already do, and much longer than patients at smaller centers. He also believes that those on other lists, particularly at units that have only recently opened, will not get as good medical treatment as they would at UCSF. Of course, he didn't say *that* at the regional meeting.

The most creative, impatient, and entrepreneurial among waiting families will organize campaigns to raise funds, pressure insurance carriers, lobby legislators, appear on "Donahue," plead with the White House—anything to get Baby X to the top of the list. And despite UNOS's oversight, it still might work, particularly if Baby X is cute, "mediagenic," and has already had one more transplant than Baby Y.

It is unlikely, however, that anyone will ever be able to duplicate a textbook media manipulation that took place in 1982. Jamie Fiske, a one-year-old liver patient, was close to the end. Her father, Charlie Fiske, combining his skills and connections as a hospital administrator with his daughter's "adorable" face, mounted a massive nationwide campaign and found Jamie a new liver in Utah. While the whole world watched, Jamie was saved from the clutches of death by a brilliant young surgeon in Minnesota named Nancy Ascher, the first woman in the world to transplant a human liver. Interestingly enough, Charlie Fiske, who has since become a board member of UNOS, admits that he manipulated the system. But he says that that is "an indictment of the system," not of himself. And the system he indicts is "the healthcare system," not the organ procurement system.

Many waiting patients are hospitalized—not all terminal, but too sick to go home. A few of the less critical are housed in residences that have been built by charitable organizations near some of the major transplant clinics. At UCLA a family or two may be found in a Winnebago camped in the hospital parking lot. Those healthy enough and close enough to the hospital to stay at home, close to beepers and phones, are hoping for these magic words: "We have a heart for you" or "Can you bring your daughter in today? We found her a liver."

The critically ill among the waiting fill pretransplant intensive care units, where specially trained nurses and physicians help them fight the last terrible battles of end-stage organ disease. They are called "status 9" patients at most hospitals, and when their physicians believe they are twelve to twenty-four hours from death, they are classified "UNOSTAT" in the UNOS computer, which places them at the top of the national waiting list.

One occasional abuse of the UNOS system has involved the questionable posting of UNOSTAT patients. UNOS officials have observed that some UNOSTAT patients remain on the list for two weeks or more, indicating that perhaps their condition was not quite so serious as it seemed. Although UNOS officials suspect some centers of exaggerating the condition of patients to get organs, they have neither the resources nor the inclination to inspect institutions and determine the status of each patient for themselves—not that it would be particularly desirable to have federal beaurocrats making unannounced site visits to diagnose terminally ill patients. But if UNOSTAT patients are going to be favored above all others, even those who could make better use of an organ, a way has yet to be found to prevent abuse. Centers caught breaking UNOS rules and procedures are threatened with fines, even suspension of Medicare funding. But when there is no way to detect an infringement, such penalties seem moot.

Amy Peele used to be the chief transplant coordinator for the University of California, San Francisco. She and other coordinators do not believe that UNOS by itself can or should solve all the problems of organ procurement, particularly in parts of the country like New York, Denver, and the San Francisco Bay Area, where rivalry used to be particularly intense and where feelings still run high among organ procurement personnel and transplant surgeons. Abuses of the system will persist, some reformers feel, until there is a stronger surveillance and enforcement apparatus either within or adjacent to UNOS. The old network "will not dismantle itself," says Peele, still a leader in the struggle for equitable distribution. "They have had it their way from the beginning, and some of them aren't going to give up their power without a fight."

Dr. Nancy Ascher, now chief of liver transplantation at UCSF and herself a partisan for sharing, describes it best. "When a surgeon accepts a patient, she makes a contract with him and his family to do all in her power to save that patient and keep him alive." This contract, Ascher points out, frequently conflicts with whatever fairness is built into the system. The force of a few hundred committed surgeons, all desperately seeking organs for their own dying patients, will always make it difficult, Ascher says, for UNOS, organ procurement agencies, or anyone else to apply the equitable ideals of national organ sharing. Ultimately the impetus for reform, she adds, must come from the public, upon which the transplant community is so much more dependent than in any other field of medicine. And it will be cases like Baby Jesse's that stimulate public interest in reform.

Jesse Sepulveda was born in 1986 with left ventricular hypoplasia, a fatal congential heart condition that is treated either with a series of palliative operations or with a complete heart transplant. He was also born out of wedlock to a seventeen-year-old mother.

When he was brought to Loma Linda University Medical Center in southern California, chief pediatric heart surgeon Leonard Bailey agreed that Jesse should be transplanted, but the Seventh Day Adventist hospital refused to admit him because his parents were unmarried, undereducated, and of questionable emotional stability. Jesse's parents took their story to the local chapter of the National Right to Life Committee, which mounted a nationwide campaign of indignation against Loma Linda and Bailey. Jesse's right to life was being denied, the committee said. The hospital should consider only that and not the social worth of his parents. When Baby Jesse's grandparents said they would raise him if he lived, Loma Linda and Bailey agreed to proceed with the transplant.

By that point, Baby Jesse was a household word in America—and a household face. In the week that led up to his transplant, he was front-page and top-of-the-morning news. His parents, therefore, had no difficulty getting scheduled on "Donahue" to tell their story and plead for Jesse's heart. While they were on the air, a phone call came in from a Frank Clemenshaw, whose newborn baby had recently died in Wyoming, Michigan. They would send the respirated body of their brain-dead son out to Loma Linda and donate his heart to Jesse. After a dramatic cross-country flight, Baby Frank's tiny heart was removed and sewn into Baby Jesse. With the whole country watching, Baby Jesse was released from the hospital with his parents (not his grandparents) about three weeks after the operation.

Several issues, medical and ethical, surfaced in the Baby Jesse case. First was the question of whether parentage and legitimacy should be considered in transplant recipient selection. This became such a hot topic in the transplant community that Loma Linda University felt compelled to sponsor a national conference on the question: Should social worth be considered in selecting patients for transpantation? Conferees let Loma Linda partly off the hook by agreeing that family support or parental competence could, in some cases, be considered a *medical* as well as social consideration, particularly when a young child was going to be reliant on the intelligent home administration of a fairly complex immunosuppressive regimen.

The second, and perhaps larger, question dealt with whether or not it was fair for the family of a dying patient to appeal directly to the public for a scarce commodity. The Sepulvedas had successfully bypassed the official organ procurement network. Transplant coordinators and organ procurement officials were furious, particularly when they learned that a specific child,

Baby Calvin of Louisville, Kentucky, who was next in line for the heart that Jesse got, almost died. (Calvin got a heart a few days later and survived his transplant.)

The transplant community knows that almost any dramatic story about successful organ transplanting is good for its cause. But transplant coordinators believe that that will be the case only if the Baby Jesse incident is remembered not as a heroic surgical rescue but as a case of systemic abuse.

NATIONAL RESOURCES

Once Jacesohn Walden's organs were removed they became, according to the National Task Force on Organ Transplantation that conceived UNOS, a "national resource." They were, in theory at least, the common property of the American people (as opposed to the personal property of a survivor, beneficiary, or surgeon). If the system was working as designed, each organ would ultimately go to the closest potential recipient with the best blood and tissue match. If there was more than one potential recipient that fit that description, the appropriate organ would go the person that had been waiting the longest.

Unfortunately, despite the arrival of a new regimen, the organ-as-national-resource theory remains just that—a theory. An organ is still, de facto, the property of the center that harvests it. And while the selection of that team is now most often made on a strict rotational basis by a regional organ procurement agency, property registered with UNOS, the final choice of a recipient remains the privilege of surgeons and committees in the transplant units.

The selection of recipients for Jacesohn's heart, liver, kidneys, and corneas was, in fact, an eclectic mix of UNOS-mandated practices and conservative medical traditions. Although there was no impropriety in the final selection of any recipients, the processes revealed residues of the old network.

It seems unlikely that distribution of organs will ever be truly fair as long as there are ways that a Charlie Fiske or a Jesse Sepulveda can manipulate or bypass the system. Until the chronic shortage of organs is somehow eliminated, waiting patients can only lie and watch—and hope that most of their fellow patients will wait their turn as well.

PART TWO

THE CHOSEN

People who suddenly lose someone very close are not always themselves for a while. They are sometimes even surprised by their own behavior.

In one instance the family of an organ donor arrived at the home of a recipient on the donor's birthday. They wanted to hold a small celebration in the proximity of their loved one's liver. In another incident a woman turned up at a heart recipient's front door with a stethoscope. For "just one last time" she begged to hear her husband's heartbeat. Recipients have even received invoices from donor families charging them for the organ that saved their lives.

Recipients, too, have at times, with the best of intentions, made life harder for the survivors of organ donors. Some become so guilty about gaining life from another's death that they are unable to resist writing or calling donor relatives, often exacerbating their grief.

It hasn't always worked out badly when recipient meets donor family; there have been some wonderful bonds and friendships formed. But they appear to be exceptional. Psychiatrists and social workers who attend to transplant patients and their families have come to believe that it is better if recipients are not aware of their donors' identity and vice versa.

Transplant coordinators, hospital social workers, and surgeons, who are usually the first to discover the *consequences of their work, were without exception willing to talk openly about the medical and psychological aspects of each case involving the recipients of Jacesohn Walden's organs, but with the stipulation that the identity of recipient patients not be revealed. Although it is unlikely that the Waldens (their real name) would behave in any but the most respectful and sensitive way, the names, hometowns, and clearly identifiable facts about the people who were chosen to receive Jacesohn's organs have been changed.*

CHAPTER 4

KIDNEY

*The challenge of transplantation is not in the operating
room, it is in the laboratory.*

NANCY ASCHER, M.D.,
University of California, San Francisco

Later on the same day, after his meeting with Lisa Tulman,
Nick Feduska decided who of the three patients he had placed
on the short list would receive Jacesohn's kidneys. His first choice
was Olivia Hernandez. For Olivia it might mean the end of a
long and tiresome ordeal with illness that had begun four years
earlier. For Feduska it meant preparing for an operation he had
performed hundreds of times. In this case, he'd be subjecting
Olivia to her *second* transplant operation.

In February 1984 Olivia Hernandez was her family's sole
provider. Her father had been injured on the job ten years before
and had been unemployed ever since. Her younger sister couldn't
find work and her mother was raising four other children and
running their small truck farm near Fresno, California.

One day, on a break from her job at a local canning factory,
Olivia noticed that her urine was the color of cinnamon. She had
not been feeling well for the previous few days, but thought it
was just fatigue. She went to the company infirmary, where a
nurse took a urine sample and sent it to the local hospital for
routine tests. The following day Olivia's supervisor approached
her on the assembly line: "Olivia, the company doctor wants to
see you right away."

Olivia walked slowly to the infirmary. There had been something in his tone that seemed ominous. "I wasn't sure I wanted to hear what the doctor had to tell me," she would remember.

When she arrived at his office, the doctor said, "Olivia, the hospital found some puzzling things in your urine. They want you to go over right away for some tests." He drove her to the hospital, where she and her bodily fluids were subjected to a series of painless but troubling tests. Olivia was then told to stay at home and rest until the results were in. If there was nothing serious, she could return to work. Two days later she was called back to the hospital. She went with her father and her sister Connie.

The diagnosis was glomerulonephritis (also known as Bright's disease), the breakdown of most of the million or more tiny ball-shaped urea filters (glomeruli) in each kidney. Sometimes Bright's disease can be cured with medicine; other cases require a transplant. In either case the patient must be placed on hemodialysis until the decision is clear.

For the next eight months, three times a week, Olivia went to a clinic and for four hours was plugged into a device, about two and half times the size of a sewing machine, that circulated her blood through a series of cellophane filters. The filters removed creatinine and urea (metabolic wastes), along with excess fluids, from her blood.

The dialysis, or "artificial kidney," machine was invented in 1943 in Nazi-occupied Holland by Willem Kolff. Kolff, a brilliant Dutch engineer and medical doctor, has since pioneered several complicated medical devices, including mechanical arms, cochlear implants, and the artificial heart. Now working at the University of Utah in Salt Lake City, where he oversaw Robert Jarvik's early research on the Jarvik-5 and Jarvik-7, Kolff is often regarded as the godfather of bionic medicine.

Versions of Kolff's kidney machine, now used worldwide, have kept millions of people alive for long, productive lives; people who would otherwise have died a slow, painful premature death. There are currently about 90,000 Americans on dialysis, although not all of them have to go to one of the 1,500 dialysis centers scattered around the country. The more fortunate are able to manage their own treatment at home with a simpler technology called peritoneal dialysis.

Dialysis does not do everything the failed kidney once did, and for many kidney patients life on the machine becomes uncomfortable and depressing. The suicide rate among dialysis patients is estimated to be almost four times that of the regular population. For most, but not all, dialysis patients, the preferable treatment for irreversible kidney failure would be transplantation. If only there were enough kidneys to go around.

By early September of 1984 Olivia had gown frustrated with dialysis. It took valuable time out of her life and exhausted her for a good part of the next day. She decided to consider a transplant and was referred to the University of California, San Francisco. After another battery of tests, Nick Feduska recommended that she receive a kidney transplant.

After describing the shortage of cadaver organs and explaining the improved results he has obtained with organs from living relatives, Feduska asked Hernandez if anyone in her family might be willing to donate a kidney. He explained that a healthy adult needs only one working kidney to live a normal life. In fact, it is widely accepted by Western medical practitioners that one kidney operating at about 50% of capacity can perform all the essential blood-cleansing functions a human needs.

Olivia went home and gathered her family. While three generations of parents, siblings, nieces, and nephews sat quietly around a crowded kitchen table, she described her illness. Olivia was not comfortable asking her relatives for a kidney, so she simply repeated in Spanish what Feduska had told her in English, including all the risks that exist for a living donor (one being death). She told them there was no urgency and asked them to think and talk about it for a while. Before she went to bed that night, every member of her family had told her he or she would give her a kidney.

"That was nice," recalls Feduska, "not only for her but also for us. The more donors we have to choose from, the better our chances of finding a good tissue match.''

By running a battery of tests matching blood and lymphocyte samples from each member of the family with Olivia's own blood, the tissue-typing laboratory at UCSF was able to determine that her sister Connie was the best histological match. After being readvised of the risks involved in losing a kidney, Connie again agreed to donate one of hers to her sister.

LRDs

About a third of the kidneys transplanted at the University of California, San Francisco, are removed from living donors, most often a close blood relative of the recipient. Statistically, Olivia stood a much better chance of keeping her sister's kidney than she would a kidney taken from a cadaver. One can add 10% to 15% to the expected one-year survival rate of patients with living related donors (LRDs), raising it at UCSF to over 95%. For this reason and because there remains an acute shortage of cadaver organs, a growing number of centers are transplanting kidneys from living donors.

The case for procuring kidneys from the living is compelling. Tissue matching between blood relatives is easy and accurate. Because there is no rush to transplant, as there is with a cadaver kidney, there is time for planning, counseling, and other preoperative preparations. A transplant can be scheduled to suit everyone's convenience. But certainly the most compelling advantage of LRDs lies in the fact that the graft can usually survive with considerably less immunosuppression than it would with a cadaver kidney.

UCSF has also found that in selected cases, if they transfuse a recipient with the blood of the donor three or four times before transplanting, they achieve dramatically improved results (96% one-year survival, 88% at four years). Donor-specific transfusions

(DSTs) are not as controversial among transplanters as LRDs, but there is strong disagreement over their necessity. The debate is only less vehement because the procedure is less likely to be harmful. There is, however, a 15% to 30% risk that a transfusion of blood from a donor will sensitize the recipient by encouraging the preformation of antibodies that will attack and reject a new organ.

Despite the improved results with LRDs, the practice is one of the most quietly debated controversies in modern medicine. The issue is, in fact, fairly well contained within the transplant community, which last year harvested about 30% of the approximately 9,000 kidneys transplanted in the United States from living donors.

Nick Feduska is an outspoken advocate of both DSTs and LRDs and claims five years of extensive research that supports his position—which he will fly almost anywhere in the world to argue. When he does so, Feduska often finds himself face to face with Dr. Thomas Starzl, his one-time mentor at the University of Pittsburgh, who tells the same audience that he will no longer take organs from living donors. For years he did so, he confesses, but stopped abruptly in 1972, when he learned that some donors (not his own) had died as a direct result of kidney removal.

Starzl claims that twenty people have died worldwide as a direct result of donating a kidney. Many of them, he hastens to point out, died in "centers of genuine excellence," dispensing with the claim that they might not have received good medical attention. He calls the fact of these deaths and their number "a well-kept secret" and says that wherever they have occurred, "they have had a devastating effect on almost everyone even remotely connected to the case." Starzl admits that his figures are based partly on anecdotal information and has yet to cite specific names and cases. But he has talked to some of the surgeons involved, and reports that they were "heartbroken . . . including one whose patient died twenty-three years ago. They told me that the donor deaths represented the most terrible moments in their lifetime.''

One of the deaths Starzl has counted occurred at UCSF. The donor died with a peptic ulcer a few weeks after the transplant. "He was so eager to donate his kidney," recalls Feduska, "that he did not tell us about his history of ulcers." And Feduska felt the deep loss described by Starzl. "He wasn't one of my patients, but I can tell you I was devastated. We all were."

UCSF had done almost 1,000 LRD transplants before experiencing its first donor death. Feduska says this won't stop him. "If you look at the worldwide record of this procedure, you will find that the death rate is only six one hundredths of one percent. That's point zero, zero, zero six percent" (.0006%).

Starzl responds: "I have heard it said, and seriously, that one death every two thousand patients is a statistical nonevent. It is hard to really believe this when the death of a single well-motivated and completely healthy living donor almost stops the clock worldwide." Starzl respectfully jibes at the case for living donors. "I never saw a living donor case done at midnight. They're always at eight o'clock in morning. They're very convenient," he told a 1986 gathering of bioethicists in Boston. It is true, of course, that with LRDs there are no hassles with procurement, recipient selection, rushed preparations, appropriation of operating rooms. And the long-term survival rates with less immunosuppression, the primary measurement of transplant success, will make any transplant unit look a lot more successful than one that will not use LRDs.

"*Primum non nocere*," Starzl reminds another group; this time it's transplant surgeons gathered at Pittsburgh in March of 1987 to debate the major controversies of renal transplantation. "First do no harm"—the very essence of the Hippocratic oath. Starzl is arguing, of course, that potential harm could be being done to the donors. Even short of death, he says, they are subject to embolisms and hypertension. "Because I cannot do it in good conscience," says Starzl, "does not mean I look badly on those who do, as long as they do so with clearly informed consent. The final decision must be between the surgeon and the living donor, and between them alone."

"First do no *harm*," bellows John Najarian, chief of surgery at the University of Minnesota and an open foe of Tom Starzl, when I repeat Starzl's admonition two months later. "What kind of harm is *he* doing by transplanting a cadaver kidney that has a seventy-five percent chance of survival in someone whose histologically matched brother, sister, or parent is willing to donate?"

UNRELATED DONORS

Minnesota, UCSF, and the University of Wisconsin have all gone one step beyond LRDs and harvested kidneys from *un*related living donors. That, of course, is even more controversial than using LRDs, not only because the compelling advantage of genetic similarity is no longer present, but also because of the fear, held by some, that it will lead to the formation of an open market in human organs in which the poor might surreptitiously sell their kidneys and portions of their pancreases to the rich, posing, if need be, as a cousin or sibling.

That practice has already been reported in Europe and is commonplace in some less developed countries. In India, Indonesia, and Brazil, for example, transplanting from unrelated donors (for money) is an open and widespread practice. Almost daily one can find advertisements in Indian papers offering either to sell or to buy kidneys or corneas. In Europe many of the surgeons that once transplanted from unrelated donors stopped doing so for fear that their practice would inevitably come to resemble India's.

The University of Wisconsin is the major U.S. user of unrelated living donors. By the end of 1987 it had done thirty-seven operations, of which thirty-five grafts survived. UCSF has done five, of which three were successful.

In the United States, concern about exploitation of the poor has motivated the American Society of Transplant Surgeons, the United Network for Organ Sharing, and the Health Care Financing Administration to add the qualifier "emotionally related" to "donor" when the donor is not related by blood. That is, living donors in the U.S., if not genetically related, must be "emotionally" related to the recipient, i.e., a spouse, step-sibling, or very close friend of the family. Abuse of this guideline can lead to strict sanctions, such as expulsion from a national organization, loss of accreditation, heavy fines, or, the worst punishment of all for a large medical center, loss of Medicare reimbursements.

OLIVIA'S FIRST

On Wednesday, October 16, 1985, Olivia and Connie Hernandez arrived together at UCSF with a large family entourage. They were admitted and prepared for surgery. The family stayed in a nearby motel. As Tom Starzl might have predicted, the operation was scheduled for 8:00 the next morning.

While for some families a living-donor transplant can be a tense and trying ordeal, there was something almost festive about this one. The affection and excitement were tangible. Nurses and social workers, who are more likely to be overworked in LRD cases, were surprised by how calm and cheerful the Hernandez family was. After father, mother, siblings, and children left for the motel, Connie and Olivia laughed and reminisced late into the night.

On Thursday morning Dr. Nick Feduska and Dr. Juliet Melzer scrub together outside adjoining operating rooms. They have teamed up on LRD transplants enough times that they can talk about anything else. So they discuss the fact that Melzer is considering pancreas transplants, a new departure for both her and UCSF, which until 1988 did only kidneys. UCSF was also planning to begin liver transplants, leaving only hearts to make it a full-service transplant center. Despite the proximity of Stanford, UCSF is now planning to open a heart transplant unit.

Once scrubbed, Feduska and Melzer step into separate operating rooms. In Feduska's is Connie Hernandez, donor; in Melzer's, Olivia Hernandez, recipient. They time their separate procedures so that Olivia is open and ready at exactly the moment when Feduska removes Connie's right kidney. At 11:16 A.M. Melzer backs through the door of Feduska's operating room with a sterile stainless steel bowl in both hands. She approaches the table like Oliver Twist asking for seconds. Without a word, Feduska drops a round pink kidney into her bowl.

It takes Melzer about forty minutes to sew Connie's kidney into a small opening on Olivia's right pelvic flank. While she does so, Feduska closes Connie, stitching the final row of sutures with the finest possible thread to minimize scarring. Both operations finish at about the same time.

By the time Feduska has dressed, dictated a detailed description of the operation over the phone to a secretary, and made his way to the recovery room, both sisters are awake. They are in adjoining beds surrounded by nurses and interns. Feduska stands between them, talking to one, then the other. Before long he has both their hands in his. He smiles, he touches, he explains and comforts—unusual for a surgeon, but Feduska is an unusual surgeon. The Hernandez sisters open and close their eyes as the anesthesia wears off.

"How do you feel, Connie?" asks Feduska.

"Cold," she says. He asks a nearby nurse for a blanket. When it comes, he takes it and places it carefully over his patient. "That better?"

"Yes," she says. "Gracias."

THE ENEMY WITHIN

No sooner had she awakened than Olivia's new kidney received some hostile visitors: killer T lymphocytes.

A subset of her own white blood cells that recognize antigens (foreign proteins) when they enter (or are placed into) the body, killer T cells join with other agents of immunity to launch a swift and vicious attack against any intruder, whether it be a virus, bacteria, parasite, piece of asbestos, or someone else's kidney. Through a microscope the "cascade" of immunity seems chaotic, but the response is actually a well-orchestrated and highly complex web of interactions at the cellular level of Olivia's body.

The purpose of the immune system is to kill microorganisms, fight cancer, and remove debris. Although there are many ways in which the system responds to invasion, all responses have one thing in common. A threat is distinguished from normal tissues by the antigens on the wall of each foreign cell. The response varies with the nature of each antigen, but it is usually swift and determined.

When Connie's kidney was sewn into Olivia's body and the vascular clamps were removed, allowing new blood to flow through it, all seemed well. The new organ turned a healthy pink and began performing its appointed functions almost immediately.

Almost all new organs do that. Kidneys pass urine, hearts begin beating, pancreases produce insulin, and livers begin to perform their metabolic functions. Even under the microscope, cellular activity seems normal for a day or two. But from the very moment that Olivia's blood touched the new kidney, small fragments of it entered her bloodstream. When the particles reached a nearby lymph node or her spleen, they were quickly identified by T cells as foreign antigens (the "T" stands for thymus, where the cells originate. B cells, the other major lymphocytes in the immune system, originate in bone marrow).

At about the same time, other T cells, called "helpers," that cruise the bloodstream looking for trouble, discovered the invader. The antigens on the kidney donated by Connie triggered Olivia's helper T cells to secret a chemical that stimulated larger immune cells called macrophages. These in turn, released a lymphokine (growth-factor protein) called interleukin 2. (Although it is believed that interleukin 2 may kill some cancer cells, its roll in graft rejection is to stimulate the production of more T cells, which rush back to the thymus to report their findings.) Each alerted T cell immediately recruited a separate platoon of polysyllabic killers—macrophages, tissue mast cells, phagocytes, and polymorphonuclear leukocytes—and dispatched them to destroy the foreigner in their own separate ways.

Each killer T cell, for example, attached itself to a target cell and injected it with a toxin called ''perforin,'' which caused holes to form in the cell wall. The punctured cell then leaked its vital fluids and died. When a few million cells had been destroyed this way, Olivia began to run a fever and show an abnormally high white cell count, very much as if she were fighting an infection (although there were no bacteria involved).

If this miraculous process, designed to protect each of us from thousands of diseases, had not been contained, it would have caused serious wreckage to Olivia's new kidney in a matter of hours. In a few days all cellular function in the graft would have ceased altogether, and eventually it would have shrunk to a useless lump of scar tissue. And the stronger Olivia's immune system was, the faster it would wreck her body's life-saving gift—an ironic and rare disadvantage of good health.

There are really only three ways of combating the rejection response. One is to place the graft in a privileged position so that antibodies cannot reach it. Another is to alter the graft itself so that it is no longer regarded as antigenic (foreign). The third method is to manipulate the immune system of the host so that it does not manufacture antibodies that will attack the graft. As transplantation has evolved, it has been the third approach that has been most successful, although recent experiments with animals has shown some success with genetic alteration of a donor organ during the ischemic period between donor and host.

Olivia's postoperative treatment required her to take three separate drugs every day: Cyclosporine, prednisore, and azathioprine. The combination was designed to suppress her immune system just enough so that it would tolerate her new kidney, but not so much that she would be vulnerable to cancer or viral diseases. It was not an easy balancing act and required her to go into a Fresno clinic for frequent blood and urine tests and to stay in regular touch with Nick Feduska.

In December of 1986, about fourteen months after her transplant, she began to grow tired and listless. Her routine tests found a high creatinine (nitrogen) level in her urine—not a good sign. It meant that her kidney was not processing nitrogen properly. A biopsy showed that her body was rapidly rejecting the organ despite the drugs she had taken faithfully every day.

Feduska increased her dosages and put her back on dialysis. When two months later she returned to UCSF for a thorough examination, Nick Feduska and his colleagues discovered to their dismay that she had completely rejected her sister's kidney and in the process of doing so had formed a lot of new antibodies. She was, he told her, "highly sensitized" and would therefore almost certainly reject any new kidney she received through a second transplant operation. Feduska, who was reluctant to remove another kidney from a family member, promised to watch for a close tissue match among the cadaver kidneys he was retrieving and to call her if he found a good one. In the meantime, she would remain on dialysis, just as she had before her first transplant.

OLIVIA'S SECOND CHANCE

In a small anteroom off the main transplant operating room at UCSF, Nick Feduska proudly shows off the kidneys he has stayed up all night to retrieve from Jacesohn Walden. They are inside a small plastic box set atop a square blue machine that pumps a refrigerated, carefully balanced preservative through each organ. The gentle, pulsing motion of the pump gives each kidney an eerily lifelike appearance.

The machine, known to some as the Belzer-Kountz system, was invented and developed in a room not far from OR 6 by America's first black transplant surgeon, Sam Kountz, who died tragically of a tropical disease following a 1974 trip to Africa, and Folkert "Fred" Belzer, a first-generation transplanter, still practicing at the University of Wisconsin. Belzer is today one of the world's leading pancreas transplanters, and an important role model to Nick Feduska. Of course, to a transplanter, anyone who has extended the ischemic time for a human organ is a hero of sorts.

Earlier that morning, Nick Feduska made his final choices from the three candidates he and Lisa Tulman had already selected as possible recipients for one of Jacesohn Walden's kidneys. First came Olivia Hernandez. As soon as he had decided, he dialed the phone.

"Olivia, this is Nick Feduska at UCSF. How are you?"

"Not so good, Doctor. I am so tired after dialysis I can hardly work. I am afraid I am going to lose my job." She was on the verge of tears.

"How would you like a new kidney?" Feduska asked in his firm but friendly voice.

"Oh, Doctor, I would be so happy," she replied.

"Can you come up today? I have an operating room scheduled for three this afternoon."

"I'll be there," she said, and arrived about 1:30 with her mother, father, two sisters, and a nephew.

By 3:15 Olivia lies anesthetized on a table in an operating room close to the perfusion machine that contains Jacesohn's kidneys. Chief transplant OR nurse Jane McIntire, who has attended at least half of the 2,800 kidney transplants performed at UCSF, teaches a young student nurse and an intern a fine point or two while they wait for Feduska to scrub. "Dr. Feduska will call these 'DeBakes,' after Michael DeBakey," she says, holding up an unusually large forcep. "It's kind of a nickname that some surgeons use; but not all. You will never, for example, hear Dr. Shumway call them 'DeBakes.' " She laughs, but the joke is over the heads of students too young to remember the deep rivalry that once existed between DeBakey and Norman Shumway.

FIRSTS

There are several claims to the first "successful" kidney transplant. They originate in Europe and North America, and the rivalry is intense. Since there has never been an adequate definition of success, one is tempted to conclude that they all deserve the honor. Certainly, one of the most amusing early transplants was performed in 1947 at Boston's Brigham and Women's Hospital by Drs. Richard Hufnagel and David Hume.

One night while he was working late in the surgical research lab at Harvard, Hufnagel was approached by a urologic resident named Ernest Landsteiner. Landsteiner had a very sick patient with kidney failure. She was, in fact, anuric (without urine) and about to die. Would Hufnagel be interested in transplanting a cadaver kidney to tide her over long enough to get well? Hufnagel agreed to try and dispatched his friend Hume to find a cadaver. Hume found a suitable donor the same day.

"Because the patient was extremely critical," recalls Hufnagel, "there was some administrative objection to bringing her into an operating room. So, about midnight, when the kidney had been removed from the donor, our little group (Landsteiner, Hume, and myself) proceeded to an end room on the second floor and, by the light of two small gooseneck student lamps, prepared to do the transplant." Together, the three young surgeons transplanted the cadaver kidney into the upper arm of their moribund patient. Although they were unable to completely enclose the kidney in the patient's skin, to their surprise and joy it immediately began to secrete urine.

"Needless to say, we hovered closely about for a considerable number of hours," recalls Hufnagel. "As the light of the morning dawned, our duties called us to more routine and mundane things. The kidney continued to excrete urine, and by noon of the next day the patient herself began to show marked improvement. She began to become more alert and by the following day was entirely clear in her mind."

The day after, with the patient showing greater improvement and with urine output declining, the team decided to remove the new kidney. About two days later she began passing urine from her own kidneys. Eventually she recovered completely.

Although the transplant had worked only temporarily, that was all it was ever intended to do. Since the patient recovered, this must certainly be recorded as a first *and* a successful transplant; if not "*the* first successful kidney transplant," it could perhaps be listed as the first nonmechanical dialysis.

Another transplant first occurred in December of 1952, after a sixteen-year-old carpenter named Marius Renard fell from a scaffolding in Paris and ruptured his right kidney. The kidney was permanently damaged and had to be removed, at which time it was discovered that he had no left kidney. This meant that the young Renard had no renal function. He, too, was anuric and would die in a few days. As his life slipped away, his mother begged the famous nephrologist Professor Jean Hamburger (the man who gave the word "nephrology" to medicine) to take one of her kidneys and transplant it into her son.

By this point, the findings of modern geneticists had convinced Hamburger that the tissues of relatives were likely to be more compatible than those of nonrelatives. On Christmas night of 1952 two of Hamburger's lead surgeons performed what was, if not "the first successful kidney transplant," certainly the first LRD transplant in history. Three weeks after the operation, young Marius was well and ready to go home, when suddenly his kidney was attacked by what would today be recognized as acute rejection. He died the next day. Although the results seem disappointing by today's standards, twenty-two days was an eternity at the time and confirmed to the medical world that genetic kinship offered at least a degree of tolerance.

The following year in Paris, Professor René Küss, now president of the Académie de Médecine, transplanted another kidney from a living related donor. That graft survived for only twenty days before rejection and seemed to indicate that while inborn tolerance definitely contributed to graft survival, it wasn't enough. Something else had to be found to suppress the tenacious human immune system.

Encouraged by Küss's and Hamburger's results, David Hume selected a twenty-six-year-old physician in kidney failure whose uremic state had, among other things, compromised his immune system. Hume thought this fact alone might decrease the likelihood of rejection. After receiving a new kidney and following an extremely difficult recovery, the patient broke a new transplant record by being the first person ever discharged from a hospital with someone else's kidney. He died about six months later of high blood pressure, not as a result of graft rejection. Despite his death, the case of Dr. W was another victory of sorts because it showed that on very rare and unpredictable occasions an organ could be tolerated without immunosuppression. However, there had been enough cases of graft failure before Dr. W to demonstrate the near universality of rejection—except perhaps in identical twins, who, having derived from the same sperm and ova, probably possessed absolutely identical immune systems.

Drs. Joseph Murray, John Merrill, and Hartwell Harrison decided to test that theory by removing a healthy kidney from Donald Herrick and transplanting it into the failing body of his identical twin brother, Richard. On December 23, 1954, Merrill and his team performed the transplant that most American medical historians recognize as "the first." With no immunosuppression whatsoever, both donor and recipient survived. Richard Herrick died eight years later of a heart attack.

But very few people who develop organ failure have identical twin siblings. If transplantation was ever going to become a widespread medical practice, some common immunological ground between unrelated donors and recipients had to be either found or induced. Enter Jean Dausset, a brilliant French immunologist working with Jean Hamburger at Hôspital Necker in Paris.

Hamburger knew after Marius Renard lived for twenty-two days that the prolonged tolerance of his mother's kidney was not a chance occurrence. The fact that all the blood groups and subgroups of the son were identical to those of his mother was to Hamburger and Dausset a clue. Would it be possible, they asked themselves, to find similar genetic markers in *un*related people that would help surgeons select the right donor for a kidney? "We did the most ridiculous thing," recalls Hamburger with characteristic modesty. "We studied and compared the shapes of people's ears, the color of their eyes, their fingerprints, and many other morphological features. We took thousands of pictures hoping to find a common marker. Of course, this led to nothing."

In 1958 Jean Dausset, who had already isolated some genetic markers of human individuality, was studying the reactions between antigens and antibodies and found a leukocyte antigen that he thought might be the one responsible for graft rejections— the Mac or Group 1 antigen. Thus began an extraordinary scientific adventure that led to the discovery of human leukocyte antigens (HLA) on the short arm of the sixth chromosome.

Discovering HLA was the first critical step toward the development of the tissue-matching system that, although controversial, is still used at many transplant centers to match organ donors and recipients. Hamburger remembers that Dausset's work was regarded with great skepticism at the time. "If we may be proud of one thing in the history of transplantation," Hamburger said some twenty-five years later, "it is our stubbornness in sticking to the idea of immunologic selection of the human donor, in the face of an ocean of skepticism." For his discovery of HLA and its contribution to human tissue matching, Jean Dausset was awarded a Nobel Prize.

Being able to match organs to humans advanced the science

of kidney transplantation from experiment to treatment. Although it was a brilliant discovery that lead to other important medical realizations, including the hazard to kidney transplants from pre-formed antibodies, tissue matching was not, by itself, enough to go on.

While in many cases the ability to match donor and recipient was an invaluable addition to surgical decision making, the complexity of the immune system has made matching between un-related people more difficult than Hamburger and Dausset anticipated. If there was ever to be a meaningful number of successful transplants performed, a better way to suppress at least part of the system simply would have to be found.

During the years that followed, a combination of methods was attempted to combat rejection. In Europe and Boston pre-operative full-body irradiation was attempted with minimal success. The damage done to the immune system by the radiation was simply too debilitating. Although some scientists are still attempting to induce tolerance with radiation, they are working only with animals.

A VERY UNUSUAL CASE

Scrubbed, robed and masked, Feduska uses his hip to push open the door of the operating room in which Olivia Hernandez rests.

"Gloves, please."

A pair of surgical gloves are placed on his hands by a nurse. He begins his work with ease. While positioning Olivia's sleeping body for the operation, he explains the case to some medical students who are present:

"This patient has already been transplanted once. The kidney came from a living related donor, her sister. Six weeks after the operation, she began to reject. We increased her cyclosporine and put her on prednisone. That didn't work, so we cut back the cyclosporine and tried OKT3, a monoclonal antibody that has been found useful in acute rejection episodes. When it works, it goes right to the site of rejection and stops it. OKT3 worked for a while but we couldn't keep her on it forever. When we went back to cyclosporine and prednisone, she rejected again. So we put her back on dialysis and back on the list. This is a very unusual case. Our results with living related donors have been excellent. But every now and then they fail and we have to retransplant."

Feduska makes a short incision on the side opposite the scar from the last operation. The skin parts easily. There is little bleeding. As he proceeds with the "Bovie," an electric scalpel that cauterizes small blood vessels as it cuts down through the thin layers of fat and muscle, Feduska continues his lecture:

"Now, this patient was highly sensitized by her previous transplant. For a while after she rejected, there weren't many kidneys in the world that she wouldn't have rejected. We waited for a while until her PRA [panel reactive antibody] dropped a little, and then by removing a couple of lymph nodes from the donor, we were able to test and found them to be a much better antigen match than we would normally insist on. The donor of the kidney we have for her is, in fact, almost as well matched as Connie's was. That wasn't easy to find. She is very lucky."

"Deavers" (large retractors) are placed in the incision and the peritoneum is pulled back to reveal the last remaining site where a kidney can be placed. Her two original (nonfunctioning) kidneys remain in their original location, high in the abdominal cavity behind the liver. Her first transplanted kidney, now completely useless, sits on the right side of her pelvic region just below her appendix. Unless there is reason to believe that they are contributing to rejection or other medical problems, transplanted kidneys that fail are normally left where they are. So, for this transplant, Feduska has opened Olivia's left pelvic area and tied off the iliac vessels to which Jacesohn's kidney will be attached.

"Bring in the new kidney, please," Feduska says. The perfusion machine is wheeled in. Feduska removes the catheters from the veins and arteries of Jacesohn's kidney, which he carefully rinses in a sterile bowl. Having done so, he lays the new kidney gently inside Olivia's pelvis next to the artery and vein he has tied off. And the anastomosis (joining of vessels and ducts) begins.

Using techniques developed at the turn of the century by vascular surgeon and Nobel Laureate Alexis Carrel, Feduska sews together the delicate veins and arteries with sutures so fine they can barely be seen from three feet away. In less than half an hour the anastomoses are complete, and the key moment approaches. Vascular clamps will soon be removed from the arteries and veins leading into and from the new organ, and Olivia's blood will be allowed to flow into Jacesohn's kidney for the first time. Soon thereafter Feduska will know if it functions. The first sign: urine.

The clamps are removed. The kidney turns a vibrant pink. The room is hushed. All eyes are on the still-unconnected end of the ureter leading from the kidney. The wait is interminable. Are the kidney's million-plus ball-shaped filters doing their work, filtering the urea and other poisons from Olivia's blood, or has ischemia wrecked the kidney? Each second seems like an eternity. In less than a minute a golden droplet appears at the end of the ureter. There are sighs. The ureter spasms and a spurt of urine arcs from the wound onto the table. There are cheers. The first hurdle is cleared. The kidney has replaced dialysis.

Now the ureter must be attached to the bladder (ureteroneocystostomy), a somewhat trickier procedure than the ones that have come before it. The bladder must be opened while the ureter is sewn to the interior membrane. When the incision in the bladder is sutured up tightly, the operation is basically over.

"Okay, lets close," says Feduska, who explains to his residents that Olivia Hernandez will be more closely watched than most transplant patients. In fact, she will be watched by many in the transplant community who will follow her case through journal articles and in conversations held with her widely traveled surgeon at medical conventions, where there is often greater interest in one unusual case than in a slide show filled with bland statistics about thousands of others.

Many factors make this case unique. Olivia is a recipient from a living related donor (LRD), a retransplanted patient, a graft rejector, and a graft survivor—all in one. She has furnished the medical profession with more data than most transplant patients. Olivia's contribution to the statistics are vital.

THE ROLE OF STATISTICS

Statistics are more than a badge of honor in transplantation. They can be the lifeblood of a transplant center or even an entire practice. For it is statistics that bureaucrats watch in deciding whether to extend entitlement to a particular treatment or approval to a specific medical center for reimbursement. It is statistics that the UNOS studies before it will accept a center in the network. Survival rates are vital information to insurance actuaries, who must calculate their premiums on the basis of results. Impressive results also attract patients, talent, and prestige to an institution. Bad statistics can shut it down.

One-year survival rates for cadaver kidney transplants vary widely from one center to another. Nationwide, they are getting close to 90%. Add 5% to 10% for LRD transplants. Two-year cadaver donor rates are 75% to 80%, and five-year rates about 70%.

Second-generation transplanters like Feduska are beginning to believe that one-year rates are no longer a significant indicator of excellence. One-year rates are a holdover from the days when a graft that survived for a full year was a cause for celebration. "We shouldn't pay so much attention to one-year rates," says Feduska. "Five years give a much better indication of how well a center is doing."

With a national cohort of living kidney transplant patients

numbering in the thousands, it is now possible to determine
ten-, fifteen-, even twenty-year graft survival rates. It is at ten
years and beyond that factors like tissue matching and various
immunosuppressive regimens begin to show significantly different results. During the next decade the long-term effects of suppressing the human immune system will make themselves evident.
The results will be the clinical culmination of three decades of
research that are worth recalling before we learn how Jacesohn
Walden's second kidney and other organs were used.

ADVANCING THE ART

On June 13, 1959, a short article appeared in the British journal
Nature that signaled a possible breakthrough in immunologic
tolerance. The article was by Drs. Robert Schwartz and William
Dameshek, two relatively unknown research physicians at the
Blood Research Laboratories of Tufts University in Boston, Massachusetts. Schwartz and Dameshek described a simple experiment they had performed in which rabbits were injected with an
antigen that had been tagged with a radioactive iodide so that it
could be detected in blood samples later drawn from the rabbits.
Normal rabbits with healthy immune systems, they found, were
quickly able to remove the foreign protein from their serum. One
group, however, was also injected with 6-mercaptopurine, a drug
that was being used in the treatment of cancer, in addition to
getting an injection of the antigen. For many weeks after the
injections the rabbits were unable to reject the radioactive antigen
from their circulation. While Schwartz and Dameshek were able
only to theorize the pharmacology of this response, they were
convinced they had observed drug-induced immunological tolerance. They were right. A year later, in fact, they announced
that by using 6-mercaptopurine they were able to triple the survival time of skin grafts in the same breed of rabbits.

Within months of that report Dr. Roy Calne (now *Sir* Roy

Calne, knighted by Queen Elizabeth II in 1981), a young surgeon working at the Buckston Browne Research Farm of the Royal College of Surgeons in England, began experimenting with 6-mercaptopurine in dogs with kidney transplants. Although he had difficulty keeping his dogs alive for more than a few days post-transplant, he found that none of them were rejecting the kidney. They were dying of other causes. Since lung diseases and other postoperative problems were fairly common in dogs, Calne and the transplant community took his results as a good sign.

For the next ten years or so, 6-mercaptopurine and azathioprine (brand named Immuran) became the most widely prescribed drugs in transplantation. A combination of Immuran and corticosteroids (prednisone mostly) used in differing ratios and dosages became the regimen of choice. "Cocktail therapy," it was called, as, like the martini, the desired ratio of ingredients varied widely from patient to patient, depending on his or her immunological tastes and reactions to either of the drugs—both of which displayed unsavory and painful side effects. In 1966 a new ingredient, antilymphocyte globulin (ALG), was added to the cocktail.

ALG is made out of the antibodies formed in a rabbit, goat, or horse when the animal is injected with human white blood cells. Once the animal's immune system has created the antibodies, the animal's blood is extracted, purified, and made into an injectable serum. Known as "horse ALG" or "rabbit ALG," depending on its source, the drug is used during the first weeks or months after transplantation.

As brilliant and effective as ALG was, particularly when steroids didn't work, it still had limitations simply because it was *poly*clonal and therefore difficult to target. In 1975 in Cambridge, England, a hint of improvement appeared in the work George Kohler and Caesar Milstein, who found that when they injected hybridomas (cancer cells) into mice, they would product a *mon-o*clonal antibody (identical cells procured from a single cell) that could aim itself directly at specific immune cells.

Using Kohler and Milstein's techniques, an Australian immunologist named Gideon Goldstein, working for Ortho Pharmaceutical Corporation in Raritan, New Jersey, found that he could fuse special hybridomas to produce antibodies that would attack only the specific T lymphocytes that are the enemy of grafted tissue. While OKT3, as Goldstein named it, would not be approved for general use until 1986, it was found in clinical trials to be useful in combating acute or sudden rejection of kidneys and other transplanted organs.

OKT3 was a major breakthrough, and Kohler and Milstein won Nobels for their contribution to the development of monoclonal antibodies. But OKT3 was not a drug the human body could withstand for a lifetime. And graft rejection is not something the human body tries only once. It's a lifelong effort. By the mid-1970's there were still very few surgeons describing transplantation as a "successful" treatment. "It was almost a scandal nationwide how bad the results were with cadaveric transplantation," remembers Tom Starzl. "Expectations had been inflated . . . and very few centers had the courage to report their results," he recalls with some embarrassment. "Nephrologists who were promoting one flawed method of therapy, dialysis, were engaged in spitting contests with transplant surgeons who were inflating the expectations offered by their specialty. It was a debate hardly worth entering into, but it raged right up through the early 1980s."

A more gentle suppressor of the immune system was badly needed. A young Swiss biologist named Jean-François Borel tripped over one while looking for a new antibiotic.

THE MAGIC BULLET

Executives at the Sandoz Chemical Company in Basel, Switzerland, remembered that some of the most exciting medicines have been found in simple places like the mold on a piece of bread, the yoke of a fertile egg, or a handful of dirt. So they established a rather unusual practice that today is part of the company's basic research protocol. Sandoz scientists routinely carry soil samples back with them from any part of the world that they visit on business or vacation.

Organ transplantation was revolutionized by a few ounces of tundra soil taken in 1970 from a bleak, treeless plateau in southern Norway called Hardanger Vidda. When Sandoz chemists began their routine analysis of the soil, they found in it an unusual fungus. Tolypocladium Inflatum Gans (TIG), they named it. TIG had chemical properties suggesting that it might be used to develop either an antibiotic or an antifungal agent. Pharmaceutical companies are in constant search of such options. They are very profitable. Although tests found the materials extracted from TIG to be useful against a few strains of fungus, it was finally concluded that it had no medical value. It was labeled "Compound 24-556" and placed on the shelf.

But Jean-François Borel, a thirty-five-year-old Sandoz biologist who had studied at the University of Wisconsin, was curious about some of the chemical properties displayed by some of the compounds extracted from TIG, particularly one, a metabolite of the fungus composed of eleven amino acids hooked together in the form of a ring. This peculiar "polypeptide" suppressed the immune system of mice but did not kill cancer cells in their bodies. Borel was intrigued. "We had never seen anything like this at Sandoz," he said, and kept playing with it, pretty much on his own time.

At one point Borel injected the compound into a culture of lymphocytes. The lymphocytes, he observed, stopped growing and could barely function. However, they did not die. Additional experiments showed that the compound was able to sabotage a whole range of immune responses. Such properties had never been seen in the small pharmacopoeia of immunosuppressive drugs in use at the time. Borel purified the TIG compound and by 1974 had a substance that inhibited helper T lymphocytes from producing interleukin 2, the hormonelike agent that stimulates killer T lymphocytes.

Borel named his new compound "ciclosporin." In later trials he noticed that his new compound did not kill bone marrow cells, another unusual property for an immunosuppressive agent; nor did it act on phagocytes and thereby weaken a body's immunological response to bacterial or fungal infection. Most important, however, was Borel's discovery that when ciclosporin was withdrawn, the white blood cells it had suppressed quickly returned to full strength and continued their work as defenders of the body. This, of course, was good and bad news at once. Good news because it showed that ciclosporin did no permanent damage to the immune system and could be tapered off with positive results if the original dose proved to be too strong; but bad news because it meant that, once the optimal dose was established, people requiring the drug would have to stay on it for the rest of their lives, despite whatever side effects remained.

In 1976 Borel read a paper at a meeting of the British Society of Immunology, saying that he had observed remarkable properties in a purified compound (by then he had respelled it "cyclosporine") and that he had observed the results in mice, rats, guinea pigs, rabbits, dogs, and monkeys. A British researcher named David White carried word of this new immunosuppressive agent back to Cambridge. Sir Roy Calne, by then the most prominent transplant surgeon in Britain, asked for a sample of the compound and immediately began his own experiments with transplanted animals.

With heart transplants in pigs, the best Calne and his group had been able to accomplish was a six-day survival rate. With cyclosporine, they began to get survival rates ranging up to 200 and 300 days. Calne was so excited about the early results that he and White wrote to Sandoz asking for more of the compound. Borel wrote back to say that Sandoz had dropped cyclosporine from its research list. There was no more.

"Sandoz had never discouraged me from doing this work,"

recalls Borel, "but product championship has always been a little difficult in the company. Some people there understood what cyclosporine was, others didn't. Few thought immunology was an interesting field, particularly the money men, with whom I had the most difficulty. Fortunately, top management was fairly flexible then. They let me invite David White and Roy Calne down here to make a presentation."

Sir Roy Calne is an extremely charming and persuasive man. He convinced them that transplantation was going to become a large-scale medical practice and that cyclosporine showed promise of playing a major role. Sandoz management was impressed and agreed to produce some more. "I'm not sure cyclosporine would be discovered there today," says Borel. He remains with Sandoz but spends much of his time on the road, speaking at transplant conventions and helping other scientists improve his discovery, analogues of which are still being developed. Cyclosporine, now manufactured at Sandoz's Austrian facility, has become the company's third-largest-selling drug. In the United States it is number one.

Transplant surgeons in Europe, the U.K., and America joined Calne and began testing cyclosporine in transplanted animals. By 1978 Calne was ready to test in humans. Early results were disappointing. There was a high mortality rate and an alarming number of lymphomas (lymph cancers) in the early Cambridge clinical trials, while tests in Boston and Colorado revealed some other unsavory side effects. A 1979 article by Calne in *Lancet*, the most widely read British medical journal, reported a high cancer rate among his thirty-four test patients. "That article almost meant the end for cyclosporine again," recalls Borel. Some of those testing it in England publicly recommended that the drug be abandoned.

It became clear to Borel, Calne, and other scientists testing cyclosporine that this drug required even more careful management than the azathioprine-steroid "cocktail," and that patients taking it would have to be closely monitored for life. Tom Starzl, who was still working at the University of Colorado, began combining cyclosporine with steroids and was able to sharply reduce the dosage of both and obtain good immunosuppression. The best news, however, was a concomitant reduction in cancers among new patients.

Two years later, exuberant physicians—particularly Calne and Starzl—predicted at a symposium at the Albert Einstein College of Medicine in New York that a refined version of the wonder drug called cyclosporine A (CyA), nicknamed the "magic bullet," would change the course of modern medicine. *World Medicine*, an international health sciences journal, covered the event and reported that "cyclosporine A, it seems, is not only a valuable immunosuppressant, but can also provoke profound euphoria in transplant surgeons."

Sandoz's own clinical trials revealed, and others complained of, difficulty metabolizing the drug. But Borel experimented on himself by taking it with water, alcohol, and other liquids until he found that when he mixed it with olive oil, it would later turn up in his bloodstream. After announcing his recommendation, "I was accused of trying to poison the English," remembers Borel.

Cyclosporine or CyA (now marketed under the brand name Sandimmune) may not yet have revolutionized medicine, but it certainly revolutionized transplantation, and transplantation may yet revolutionize medicine. Today, almost every transplant patient is routinely placed on a drug regimen that includes CyA. Usually their treatment involves CyA in combination with relatively small doses of steroids or other immunosuppressants. With CyA, transplanters are now able to cross tissue barriers they could barely approach before its discovery. Thousands more people around the world have been given a second chance at life as a result.

And transplant surgeons have had a rebirth of their own. According to Starzl, "the clinical transplant sessions at scientific society meetings [held throughout the 1970s] had become tedious expositions in which claims of results, counterclaims, and shuffling of details filled the programs. The boredom was shattered with the arrival of cyclosporine.''

The transplant industry has literally boomed in the United States since November 1983, when the Food and Drug Administration finally approved CyA for general use, and with good reason. Despite some lingering imperfections, clinical studies comparing CyA to azathioprine, the most popular contemporary immunosuppressant, showed a one-year graft survival rate of 80% for CyA compared to 61% for azathioprine. It was also found that CyA could be used effectively with much lower doses of prednisone than azathioprine could.

Before CyA was cleared, liver transplantation had been abandoned at all but one small center in the U.S. With a one-year survival rate of only 32%, the procedure was still considered highly experimental. When tests with CyA raised the survival rate to 70% and the drug was cleared, most of the major transplant centers in Europe and the U.S. began to offer new livers as a regular surgical service.

Heart transplants had also been discontinued. After Christiaan Barnard's daring first in 1967, there was an ''epidemic'' of attempts that lasted into the early 1970's, but the results were abysmal and one by one the leading hospitals of the Western world suspended the procedure until tests with CyA brought one-year survival rates in most centers from under 50% to 80%.

CyA also made the combined transplant of heart and lungs possible for the first time and has had promising results in conjunction with pancreas transplantation. Heart-lung transplant pioneer Dr. Bruce Reitz says that, pre-cyclosporine, the procedure was virtually impossible ''because the drugs used then were so toxic that they knocked out every element in the immune system.''

As a tribute to cyclosporine, the convocation of the International Transplant Society in 1984 was held at Hardanger Vidda, Norway. Jean-François Borel was honored. By 1987 cyclosporine was the third-best-selling drug in the Sandoz pharmacopoeia.

As magnificient as it seems and as great as is its potential,

CyA is not a panacea. First, it is very expensive, costing between $4,000 and $7,000 a year, depending on the dose required, *for the rest of the patient's life*. The Sandoz Chemical Company says that the cost will come down when its development costs have been amortized. Market analysts predict that the price might also drop when Sandoz's patent runs out in the early 1990s and Merck, Ciba-Geigy, and others who have synthesized it enter the marketplace. Pharmaceutical history does not completely support that thesis.

CyA is also nephrotoxic (poisonous to the kidneys) in larger doses. In fact, it appears to cause some kidney problems in about 35% of all cases, and not just transplanted kidneys—*all* kidneys. It has also been linked to hypertension (increased blood pressure) in about 25% of transplant cases. And a recent report from the Mayo Clinic links cyclosporine to paralysis and seizures among liver transplant patients with extremely low cholesterol levels.

And there are less critical shortcomings. For reasons that immunologists still don't completely understand, the pace of rejection for a patient on CyA is much slower than it is for those on other immunosuppressants. Although it might seem otherwise, this is a disadvantage because it makes rejection much harder to diagnose. Most heart transplant centers perform cardiac biopsies every week for the first month or two after surgery and recommend repeat biopsies every three to four months for the rest of a patient's life. Cardiac surgeon Norman Shumway, who has by now performed more heart transplants than anyone else in the world, says that "cyclosporine is not quite the magic bullet that we had hoped it would be."

Although with smaller, more controlled doses the incidence of cancer among CyA users has dropped close to normal levels, Dr. Israel Penn of the University of Cincinnati stunned 2,000 surgeons and scientists gathered at the 1987 International Transplant Forum when he read a paper describing 239 transplant recipients who he said developed serious, although treatable, cancers that he believed were linked to cyclosporine.

The "magic bullet" (later dubbed the "penicillin of transplants") is clearly not without its problems. The FDA approval strongly recommends, although does not stipulate, careful monitoring of blood levels for all patients using the drug. CyA is nonetheless a remarkable improvement over its far more problematic predecessors—total body irradiation, azathioprine, antilymphocyte globulin, and prednisone, the side effects of which include depression of bone marrow, damage to the gastrointestinal mucosa, disturbances of sugar metabolism, osteoporosis, and Cushing's syndrome (a chronic malfunction of the adrenal glands). Unlike most of the side effects of CyA, few of these can be reduced by lowering dosages. Research is ongoing to lessen cyclosporine's side effects and improve its efficacy.

THE POST-CYCLOSPORINE ERA?

While studies focusing mostly on the molecular behavior of cyclosporine are revealing new potentials for the drug, as well as a new analogue called cyclosporine G, the quest continues elsewhere for the perfect immunosuppressant—something (like OKT3) that targets only the immune responses aimed at the new organ itself, is less expensive than CyA, has no side effects, can be tapered off to zero dosage over time, and leaves all immune cells free to fight disease or infection.

At the same International Transplant Forum where Israel Penn revealed his cancer findings, Japanese researchers announced results of tests on a new compound they call FR 900506, which like CyA inhibits the production of interleukin 2 and thereby tricks the body into accepting foreign protein. FR 900506 is about 1,000 times as potent an immunosuppressant as CyA, but Sir Roy Calne, who has tested it at Addensbrooke's Hospital in Cambridge, England, is not optimistic. "It's very toxic," he told me in London in May of 1987. "I don't think it's what we are looking for."

THE MATTER OF RACE

Frederick "Freddie" Angster, a forty-year-old telephone lineman from Sacramento, California, had been on the UCSF waiting list for over two years. Since he had been told that he was medically qualified for a transplant, he was beginning to feel that he had been passed over because he was single. Or was it, he sometimes wondered, because he was black?

There are those in the transplant community who will argue that family support, or lack thereof, is a *medical* consideration, not a "social-worth" judgment, and should therefore be considered right alongside ABO blood type and medical urgency in the final selection process.

In earlier days Stanford University Hospital made strong family support a stated prerequisite for acceptance in the heart transplant program. While it seems reasonable to assume that having plenty of loving people around to help a patient throughout a trying postoperative recovery is beneficial, several patient studies have indicated that "loners" recover just as well as those with adoring relatives, and that compliance with one's physician and medical regimen is a more important factor than family ties.

And Freddie Angster was compliant. His file in Nick Feduska's office contained letters from his personal physician and the nephrologist at his dialysis unit, both saying he was an attentive and cooperative patient. Feduska was impressed with the letters, so with a reminder from Lisa Tulman that Angster had been on the list for over two years, he gave him the nod.

Angster was ecstatic when the call came from Tulman. Although he was as compliant as his file suggested, he was also tired of dialysis. He had tried to make life as normal as possible, even traveling to Europe the previous summer after writing to kidney centers in Paris, Rome, London, and Madrid to make certain he could stop by on specific dates for dialysis. And although he was classified as "partially handicapped" by the phone company, he carefully scheduled his dialysis to avoid missing work. He had perfect attendance record. But that didn't mean he enjoyed lying still for dialysis three or four hours a day three of four times a week. Nor did he appreciate that weak, seminauseous feeling that often lasted for hours after each session.

Like Olivia Hernandez, Angster had only a few hours to be at the hospital. He called the phone company and told them he would be out sick for a couple of weeks, packed a suitcase, and jumped into the Plymouth Valiant he had kept constantly above half full for just this occasion. While the perfusion machine gently pumped a cool preservative through Jacesohn Walden's kidney, Angster cruised down Interstate 80 at a careful 55.

Although Freddie Angster had the right blood type, was compliant, and was medically suitable for transplantation, he was not that well matched, histologically, with Jacesohn Walden. Tests performed on blood samples he had left with the UCSF immunology lab showed that only three of the antigens on the short arm of his sixth chromosome matched those on Jacesohn's. That is exactly half as good as it could be—a six-antigen match. Some transplant centers might have excluded Angster from consideration. Fortunately for him, however, Feduska does not put a lot of weight on tissue matching when he selects patients for cadaver kidney transplants. In fact, he and his peers have published several papers expressing their belief that with the proper immunosuppression, matching between unrelated donors and recipients is almost irrelevant.

That, too, is a matter of serious debate among transplanters. At conventions and meetings the world over, pro-tissue-typers will precede or follow Feduska with impressive studies showing that while short-term survival rates (one to five years) are not significantly affected by tissue matching, in five to ten years after transplantation the graft survival rate is very much improved in patients with well-matched HLA (human leukocyte antigens).

Feduska won't contest the fact that in a perfect world, with an unlimited supply of kidneys, a five- or six-antigen match would improve Freddie Angster's chances of keeping Jacesohn Walden's kidney. But he argues that in the imperfect world of long waiting lists, short ischemic time, and organ scarcity, the slightly larger doses of cyclosporine that might be required by Angster should not exclude him from being transplanted with an imperfectly matched kidney.

Feduska also knows that there are small but significant differences between blacks and whites in the frequency of some lymphocyte antigens. Despite the additional complications that could arise because of this difference, about 80% of all blacks who are transplanted receive kidneys from white donors. A survey conducted by Howard University found that blacks were much less willing than whites to donate their own or their loved ones' organs after death. Ironically, the most common reason given by those surveyed was fear that whites would get the kidneys and blacks would be passed over.

The suspicion of unfairness runs deep in the black community. Clive Callender, a black transplant surgeon from Howard University, works hard to dispel fears and increase black organ donation. In articles and in a speech he makes several times a year to black audiences, Callender stresses the point that most of the organs transplanted to blacks are from whites, and makes an impassioned plea for a change of heart in his community. "Blacks aren't donating. We're taking but we're not giving back," he says. "Since we have a unique predilection for high blood pressure and kidney failure, it is even more important that blacks should become interested in doing something to help themselves." He also points out that more blacks than whites per capita suffer the kind of kidney failures that require transplantation, reminding his audiences that an improved survival rate among black transplant patients will come with the improved HLA match that is assured with black kidneys.

Angster's transplant was performed by Oscar Salvatierra, Jr., head of the UCSF transplant unit and a high-profile activist in the politically complex world of transplantation. A soft-spoken Vietnam combat surgeon, Salvatierra enjoys transplanting, but finds that speaking, lobbying, and teaching keep him farther away from the operating room than he would like. As former president of the American Society of Transplant Surgeons, an organization that has only recently gained the respect he feels it deserves in the medical community, Salvatierra lobbied for federal legislation that both regulated and protected organ transplanting. Though he enjoys discussing the politics of transplantation, he is cautious in expressing his views.

"We are moving toward a concept of designated transplant centers in this country," he tells me as we head toward the operating room where Freddie Angster is waiting for his new kidney. "In the future, only hospitals that meet rigid specifications will be cleared to practice transplantation." In the world of transplantation, with its bold initiatives and independent explorers, that is a radical idea. But like the administrators of most large transplant units, Salvatierra is becoming concerned about the proliferation of smaller centers staffed by less skilled and experienced surgeons and immunologists. He therefore supports a recent government move to set strict criteria for any hospital wishing to open a new transplant center.

"Now, that's something the AMA is strongly opposed to," he says. "Their primary advocacy is for the doctor and the maintenance of his or her practice, and the AMA rejects anything that interferes with the physician's prerogative to practice medicine the way he sees fit." Salvatierra says his own orientation is less toward his fellow physicians and more toward his patients. "The reason we got the Organ Transplant Act through the legislature was not by promoting the interests of physicians; it was pure patient advocacy."

As he scrubs his hands and forearms with iodized soap, Salvatierra explains why in 1983 he resigned his position as vice president of the American Council on Transplantation (ACT), an umbrella organization allegedly representing all aspects of the transplant community. "After I agreed to become an officer of ACT, I discovered that it had strong ties to the Reagan administration, which, of course, was opposed to the Organ Transplant

Act.'' Not wanting to be identified as part of an administration front that was opposing the same legislation he supported, Salvatierra resigned from ACT along with Amy Peele and two other members of its board. It was a devastating blow to the fledgling organization—a blow, in fact, from which it has yet to recover. ''When ACT saw the momentum behind the bill and realized that they would be the only organization representing transplantation and transplant patients that were opposed, they changed their mind at the last minute and supported it.''

The operation to give Freddie Angster one of Jacesohn's kidneys was identical to Olivia Hernandez's, except that this time the kidney was placed on the opposite side of the recipient's body.

Freddie Angster is back at work, wishing he didn't have to take so much medicine but happy to be off dialysis. Like Dr. Clive Callender, he now actively encourages blacks to donate organs for transplantation.

At last report, Olivia Hernandez had overcome one minor rejection episode, was dialysis-free, and had returned to work with Jacesohn's kidney functioning at 100% capacity. The only residual problem with her illness was a disagreement between her employer and his health insurance company about whether or not Olivia should have been placed back under the group policy with ''a pre-existing condition.'' He has promised Olivia either to fight the company or to change carriers.

CHAPTER 5

HEART

Such is the force and power of individuality, that if anyone should believe that he could accelerate and increase the beauty of union, nay more, achieve even the least part of the operation, we consider him plainly superstitious and badly grounded in physical sciences.

GASPARE TAGLIACOZZI,
Renaissance surgeon

Ralph Sanduski used to mow the lawn every Saturday morning between 11:30 and 11:50. The rhythmic drone of his faithful old Briggs & Stratton had become a mantra that kept the world away for the twenty minutes it took to groom his modest share of Denver suburbia. When the lawn was cut, he would have ten minutes left to dump the cuttings and put away the lawn mower before pouring the one prelunch martini he allowed himself every week. Although he made light of that half hour, often calling himself "Wally Weekender" when friends dropped by, it was a time of life he loved and valued. After his 1984 heart attack it was one of the few exertions he could still afford without becoming completely exhausted.

Near the end of September 1986, when most of the mowing was over in Colorado, Sanduski's cardiologist told him not do it anymore. In fact, he told him not to do anything that would make his heart beat faster—jog, swim, bicycle, make love. His heart would demand more oxygen, which it wouldn't get because the arteries that fed oxygen to muscle had hardened (arteriosclerois).

His heart would quit and he would die on the lawn or on the trail or in bed. The doctor also advised him to retire early from his work as a production supervisor at a small air-conditioning company. The only thing that would get Sanduski back to work and the lawn mower, said his doctor, was a new heart.

There is a heart transplant center in the Denver area, but Ralph's wife, Gretta, had read somewhere about Stanford University's program. The article said that Stanford, "a sort of Lourdes for people with failing hearts," had one of the best postoperative survival records in the world. Gretta believed that when it came to health, you went for the best.

"Ralph, let's drive out there and visit those folks," she said. "We could stop and see Beth and the kids on the way." Beth is the oldest of their four children and now lives in Sacramento. "What the hell," said Ralph to himself, "I'm only fifty-one years old. I don't want to live like this for the rest of my life." The truth was—and he hadn't told Gretta this—that his doctor had told him that without a transplant he might not last a year. A new heart could give him five, maybe even ten, more good ones.

After Ralph made an appointment to be "worked up" at Stanford, he, Gretta, and their two youngest children—Frank, seventeen, and Beatrice, twelve—jumped into the 1978 Fairlane that Ralph kept in mint condition and headed west to Palo Alto, California, via Sacramento, where Ralph disobeyed doctors orders by wrestling with his seven-year-old grandson, Biff. Though scolded by Gretta and his children, Ralph survived the match unscathed.

When they arrived in Palo Alto, a detailed examination of Sanduski's heart showed him to be in even worse condition than the Denver cardiologist had suspected. "Destruction of the muscle in the heart is worse than we suspected. I'm surprised you're on your feet, in fact," said Dr. Philip Oyer, who performed the endless battery of tests that resulted in Ralph Sanduski's being accepted for transplantation.

Although he was almost nine years older than the average heart recipient (42.8 years), Sanduski in many ways fit the average transplant profile. His diagnosis, myocardial infarction, is the most common condition requiring heart transplantation. He is male, as are 87.5% of living heart transplant patients. Like 73% of his fellow recipients, he is married. And he is among the 90% who are white.

Once a patient has been accepted and placed on a list, the timing of his or her transplant is an extremely delicate decision. A life-threatening operation probably should not be done while a patient still has some quality time left. On the other hand, one doesn't want to wait until he or she is so weak and sick as to be unable to withstand anesthesia or surgery. In between those extremes it would be difficult to chose the optimal time, since donors don't die on command.

Because he could still move around and take care of himself and there was no heart for him, Sanduski was allowed to leave the hospital while waiting for one that matched his size and blood type. Because Denver was too far from Palo Alto, Sanduski was told he should wait at his daughter's house in Sacramento. "Get a beeper system, stay close to home, don't exert yourself, and be ready to fly at a moment's notice" were among the many instructions he took with him from Palo Alto.

The Sanduskis drove back to Sacramento. Ralph stayed there while Gretta drove back to Denver so the children could return to school. It was a tense, cold, and boring winter in Denver. Gretta and the kids worried quietly about "Pop," who, they heard from Beth, was depressed. No one had ever seen him this way, particularly at Christmastime, when he had always been "Santa personified." Gretta knew that things were serious when Beth called one Tuesday morning to say that Ralph had declined to watch the Broncos on "Monday Night Football."

The sedentary life did not suit him. Nor was he overjoyed by some haunting statistics he had learned about Stanford—not about the success and survival rates, which were impressive enough. It was that 500 people came to the hospital every year for hearts and only two dozen ever got one. Even of the lucky few who were accepted for transplantation, Sanduski learned, two-thirds died waiting for a heart.

Many times Gretta considered calling Marguerite Brown at Stanford, just to make sure they hadn't forgotten Ralph. But she didn't want to be a pest. So on February 8, 1987, she asked the Denver cardiologist if he would put in a call. "Gretta," he said, "those people look at their waiting lists every day and again every time a heart comes along. But I'll call if it makes you feel better." It would, she said. An hour later the doctor called back and assured her that Ralph was on the list and that Marguerite Brown was thinking about him.

Brown didn't say so, but Ralph Sanduski's name had actually been mentioned only four hours earlier at a tense emergency meeting of the cardiac transplant unit. A heart had become available in New Mexico. The organ procurement agency in Albuquerque had been unable to find a suitable recipient in its region and had called Stanford while the meeting was under way. The only patient on the Stanford list who was close in size and weight to the New Mexico donor was Ralph Sanduski. As the cavity in the chest that houses a human heart is confined by lungs and ribs, it is important that a new heart be fairly similar in size to the recipient's own heart; the new heart must also have about the same pumping capacity. In both respects Sanduski was a fairly good match. But he was a different blood type.

In extreme emergencies, organs have been transplanted across ABO blood barriers, that is, between people with different blood types. The operation requires a complicated series of transfusions and is more likely than not to cause additional postoperative problems, including a higher likelihood of rejection.

Marguerite Brown listened intently as cardiologists, immunologists, and surgeons debated whether or not the Albuquerque heart should be accepted and transplanted across the ABO barrier into patient Sanduski. The room filled with tension as surgeons and scientists battled over abstractions of medicine.

Brown could think only of Ralph in Sacramento and Gretta in Denver. She was a bit disappointed, therefore, when the committee agreed that Sanduski's condition did not warrant the risks involved in giving him a heart with a blood type different from his own. He would either have to wait for a type A or become considerably sicker before Stanford would take a chance on another type.

About two weeks later another heart became available, in Bakersfield, California. This one was from a type A donor in Seattle and about the right size. But in the interim another Stanford cardiac patient, Harriet Orlan, had been moved to the transplant unit and placed on the waiting list. Orlan was also type A and about the same weight as Sanduski, but in much worse shape. In fact, she was hospitalized and declared in critical condition.

As the organ retrieval team sped to Bakersfield, three members of the selection committee convened again, this time informally, in an unoccupied office, to decide as fast as possible who should get the heart. Sanduski had been on the waiting list longer but Orlan was closer to death. Sanduski might make better use of a new heart; Orlan might last only a year after surgery but would probably die before the next heart arrived. Sanduski's financial report suggested he could pay in full. Orlan probably couldn't come up with much more than $85,000.

And there was the matter of family. Ralph Sanduski came from a close, loving, and supportive family. Harriet Orlan was divorced and estranged from her children. Should that make a difference? The attending surgeon would weigh all these factors and make the final decision.

In the earlier days at Stanford the choice would have been easier. There was a strict policy that heart recipients could have no other health problems besides their heart disease, they had to be compliant about taking medicine, and they had to have strong family ties. In recent years the university has gradually liberalized its restrictions for both donors and recipients, raising the maximum donor age from thirty-five to forty and recipient age from fifty to fifty-five, and accepting patients with a higher risk of failure. When Norman Shumway recently accepted a sixty-three-year-old patient for transplant, one of his colleagues quipped that "as the old man gets older, the topside limit gets higher." Stuart Jamieson, a former protégé of Shumway's who now heads the heart transplant unit at the University of Minnesota, admits that there had been rigid rules for patient selection at Stanford, but defends his mentor by pointing out that patient selection is integral to the art of transplanting. "Selecting the patients most likely to live is part of the skill," says Jamieson. "You are not doing *anyone* a favor if you waste a donor heart on someone who is going to die soon after you transplant it."

Sharp contrasts in selection policy exist from center to center. At the University of Pittsburgh, for example, which contains the country's most active transplant unit, the policy is to save the most critically ill, no matter what their age. One of the most widely discussed operations Tom Starzl has ever performed was the transplant of a liver into a seventy-six-year-old woman. At the University of Minnesota, the second largest transplant center in the country, the use of an organ is given almost as much consideration as the future of a patient. There, John Najarian, Minnesota's chief of surgery, might ask (out of earshot of the patient, of course) why such a scarce resource should go to a seventy-six-year-old when it could probably be put to better use by a fifty-year-old with the same disease. "What matters," says Richard Simmons, formerly Minnesota's chief kidney transplant surgeon and now chief of surgery at Pittsburgh, "is that we do not waste organs." That policy can mean that the least sick patients on waiting lists are more likely to be selected.

As long as organs are scarce, it seems likely that Simmons's philosophy will prevail in the American transplant community and that people like Shumway will sometimes be accused by their peers of transplanting the healthiest patients to improve their records. In Shumway's case, such an accusation doesn't seem quite fair.

The Bakersfield heart would be at Stanford in less than three hours and the chosen patient would have to be on the operating table. Sanduski was almost two hours away. There are no minutes or details of the meeting held that day, nor can we ever be privy to details of the discourse. Physicians and health workers are not anxious for patients and their families to know their positions on such difficult choices. But after an intense fifty-five minutes Marguerite Brown received a call from Norm Shumway.

"Prep Mrs. Orlan for surgery," was all he said. Ralph Sanduski would have to wait.

THE CALL

Late on the morning of March 2, 1987, as the crocuses in Gretta Sanduski's Denver garden were peeking through the last traces of a spring snowstorm, the phone rang. It was Ralph. But Gretta didn't recognize his voice. He was talking too fast.

"Honey, it's me, Ralph." He was exuberant. Marguerite Brown had just called, he said. She had found him a heart. There would be a helicopter in Sacramento in an hour and a half to take him back to Palo Alto. Gretta grabbed the suitcase she had already packed and called upstairs: "Frank it's time to drive me to the airport. Your father's on his way to Stanford."

As Gretta Sanduski cruised at 33,000 feet, gazing down at the snowcapped Sierra Nevada, Sam Walden stood by his son's bedside for the last time. If all went well, Ralph Sanduski would be on an operating table at Stanford when Marguerite Brown arrived with her picnic cooler. Despite some choppy weather in the San Joaquin Valley between Sacramento and Palo Alto, the trip went off without a hitch.

At 4:15 P.M., Norm Shumway opened the cooler and examined its contents. "Looks good," he said. "Let's put it in."

It takes a team of seven people—three surgeons, two nurses, an anesthesiologist, and a heart-lung perfusionist—about three hours to transplant a human heart. Shumway had done it more times than he could remember when he opened Ralph Sanduski. The procedure, or "protocol," he developed himself and used that day is now copied by most of the world's heart transplanters.

Through trial and error on literally hundreds of dogs, Shumway discovered that transplants worked best when the entire heart was not removed from the recipient. Now, instead of severing the major vessels, he leaves them intact, making his incision across the atria (the top collecting chambers of the heart). He then "tailors" the new heart to fit the old atria and sews it in.

It's a relatively simple operation—easier, for example, than the more common bypass and open-heart techniques. Yet despite its simplicity, one cannot deny the drama of seeing a beating heart stopped, removed, and, with a few dozen sutures, replaced with a gray bag of muscle that has been sitting in a ice bucket for four hours. The new heart lies limp and dead until clamps are removed from the great vessels surrounding it and the warm blood flows in.

Within seconds Jacesohn Walden's strong, healthy teenage heart is beating again. With luck it will continue for five or, in Sanduski's case, maybe ten more years. Over the next hour, as Jacesohn's heart gains strength and an easy rhythmic pace, its new owner is slowly weaned from the heart-lung machine. In another forty minutes he is closed and wheeled to Recovery.

BOLD VENTURES

There are two historical perspectives that can be applied to Ralph Sanduski's operation. One draws on 2,200 years of medical history, the other on 22 years of competitive research, experimentation, trial and error, controversy, and high drama. Both are relevant, of course, but Norman Shumway is a product of the shorter history.

Although not as well known as Christiaan Barnard, Denton Cooley, or Donald DeBakey, Shumway is, in fact, considered by most in the field to be the most valuable player in the human heart transplant league. He doesn't very often do transplants anymore, except on very young infants. But on this day he happened to be in the hospital and the regular surgeon on duty was not; a nice break for Ralph Sanduski.

Perspectives on transplant history vary considerably depending on which side of the Atlantic Ocean you're on. There is a persistent rivalry between Europe and North America over who did what first, where the great advances in transplantation took place, and who should have won some of the Nobel prizes for medicine that now reside in Europe. Minnesota's John Najarian chuckles with amusement at the suggestion that Jean Hamburger did the first significant kidney transplant, while Nobel Laureate Jean Dausset unabashedly describes France as the apex of world transplantation.

Actually, both Najarian and Dausset will concede that some of the most important breakthroughs in organ transplantation came from collaboration and communication between European and American scientists, such as Alexis Carrel and David Guthrie, Jean Dausset and Felix Rapaport, or Thomas Starzl and Roy Calne, and that while the early Nobel Prizes in immunology and histology rightfully belong to Europe, the next round of transplantation awards will probably go to the American and Canadian surgeons who have put European advances to such good use.

The history of medicine is replete with amusing transplantation anecdotes, some mythical, some comical, most apocryphal. There are Chinese tales of a second-century B.C. surgeon Pien Ch'iao, who allegedly swapped the hearts of two human patients; and the landmark feat of Damien and Cosme, fourth-century A.D. Cilician saints, who transplanted the leg of a black man to a wounded nobleman—an operation that was recorded by countless medieval painters. Tales abound of attempts to graft ears lost in duels, reconstruct noses destroyed by syphilis, and transplant corneas, skin, and testicles. But it was not until the early twentieth century that organ transplants as we know them began in earnest. Felix Rapaport, editor of the leading journal in the field, *Transplantation Proceedings*, identifies the collaboration of Chicago physician David Guthrie and French vascular surgeon Alexis Carrel as the starting point of modern transplant history. Carrel himself seems to have sensed the consequences of his work. After successfully rejoining the delicate veins and arteries of a thyroid gland, he wrote in 1901, "Though a simple operative curiosity today, the transplant of a gland may someday have a practical application."

In the years that followed, Carrel and Guthrie would perform what medical historian John Saunders calls "some of the most remarkable transplants of tissues and organs in the history of medicine." In 1905 they were testing some suturing techniques on a dog. Here is how they described what happened:

The heart of a small dog was extirpated and transplanted into the neck of a larger one. . . . The circulation was re-established through the heart about an hour and fifteen minutes after cessation of the beat. Twenty minutes after re-establishment of the circulation the blood was actively circulating in the coronary system. . . . Afterward contraction of the auricles appeared and about an hour after the operation contractions of the ventricles began. The heart beat at a rate of 88 per minute.

Although the dog lived for only about two hours, historians accept this experiment as the first recorded incidence of a heart separated from its blood supply being sewn into a second animal and recovering sufficiently to pump blood again.

When in 1912 Carrel received the Nobel Prize for his advances in vascular surgery, the award was strongly protested by Guthrie and his American colleagues, who claimed Carrel could not have succeeded without the collaboration of his American counterpart and had deliberately neglected to acknowledge Guthrie's contribution. True or not, Carrel and Guthrie had given medicine the suturing techniques required to transplant an organ from one being into another. And Norman Shumway used essentially the same suturing methods eighty-five years later when he stitched Jacesohn Walden's heart into Ralph Sanduski. And although it was Shumway who turned Carrel and Guthrie's methods into the recognized protocol for heart transplants, it was not Shumway who applied it first with humans.

That controversial honor belongs to a flamboyant forty-five-year-old South African cardiologist named Christiaan Barnard.

Barnard came to the United States in the mid-1960s to observe Richard Lower experimenting with dogs at the University of Minnesota. Lower had developed his technique while working with Shumway at Stanford. Today, some see Barnard as one of the great medical heroes of the twentieth century; others consider him a dangerous opportunist. The former opinion tends to originate in the media, the latter in medicine. Dr. Felix Rapaport, for example, the leading American historian of transplant medicine, describes the operation Barnard performed on December 3, 1967—when the beating heart of a brain-dead twenty-five-year-old woman named Denise Darvall was removed and transplanted into a fifty-four-year-old grocer named Louis Washansky at Groote Shuur Hospital in Cape Town, South Africa—as "one of the lowest points in transplantation history."

But that transplant, at the time dubbed "The Miracle of Cape Town," showed the world what could be done. It awakened us to the potential of a new medical technology. "True enough," says Felix Rapaport, "but it was too early. Medicine wasn't ready for it. Barnard took everything he had learned from Shumway and Lower and took it back to the only country in the world where you could take a beating heart out of another human being and did a human transplant." At the time, the country's law simply said that a person was "dead when certified dead" by a physician. In contrast, U.S. state laws then had more rigid and detailed definitions of death.

Although Washansky lived for only eighteen days, his transplant led (according to Rapaport) to "an epidemic" of premature transplants. In 1968, in fact, 101 heart transplants were performed in twenty-two countries—most of them, Stuart Jamieson recalls, "at hospitals where you would hesitate to have a simple open-heart procedure done." In the U.S. it was Denton Cooley, the "no-nonsense heart man" from Houston, Texas, who stepped in front of the camera after performing twenty-two transplants and told the world that the secret to good heart transplanting was to "cut well, tie well, and get well."

The modest and media-shy Shumway knew that Cooley was

naive, and he quietly pointed out that "the problems [with heart transplants] come *after* the surgery." Two years later only 23 of the 166 people who had been transplanted worldwide were alive, and all of Cooley's patients were dead. *Life* magazine called the whole adventure "a medical failure." One cardiologist who tried a few transplants even confessed to *Life* that he felt like he had committed "a small-scale crime against humanity." Barnard did not go quite that far, but he did admit that he and his colleagues should probably slow down a bit and study the rejection response. He also denied that he had stolen either the technique or the thunder from Shumway or Lower; in fact, he has credited Lord Brock, a British surgeon, with developing the techniques that he employed at Groote Shuur. While there was not exactly a world-wide moratorium on heart transplants, the numbers declined for a few years, and some major hospitals, like Boston's Massachusetts General, which had one of the top cardio-surgical units in the U.S., publicly announced that under no circumstances would their surgeons try the procedure.

Shumway continued his research, concentrating on the immunologic considerations that are the real challenge of the art. He did perform occasional transplants on carefully selected human patients. As a result of his caution, Stanford has built the best survival record in the world and thereby earned its reputation as the Lourdes of heart transplanting. The hospital boasts an 80% one-year survival rate, with 65% living two years and 50% more than five years.

Not everyone in transplant medicine believes that is laudable. In his autobiography, Christiaan Barnard, still the lay hero of organ transplantation, suggests that Shumway's criteria were too selective. That opinion is shared by other surgeons and continues to haunt the most successful heart transplanter in the world, i.e., that his success is due not to his brilliant surgery and postsurgical care but to the ultraconservative selection of patients.

Shumway is easier on Barnard than Rapaport is: "It's very important for Chris to have a celebrity status." (Richard Lower, who admires Barnard's courage, says, "It took a lot of guts.")

Shumway is also remarkably undefensive about his own practice and accepts his limited fame. "Who remembers the second man to reach the North Pole?" he once quipped. Twenty years and over 200 successful transplants later, Shumway simply says, "I know who I am, and those who are conversant with the field know too. The greatest thing you can have is the respect of your peers."

People who work with Shumway are less generous with Barnard. "The politest thing I can say about him is that he is an opportunist," says Marguerite Brown, who has worked at Stanford's cardiac unit for twelve years. In response to Barnard's remark about Shumway, she responds, "That's ridiculous." In response to the idea that Shumway selects his patients to protect his own record, she explains that "we regularly take patients that no one else will transplant." Harriet Orlan is an example.

THE ULTIMATE BATTLE

"Taking a heart from a cadaver and attaching it to a new body is actually a rather simple procedure," admits the strong-willed John Najarian. "I could teach an intern to do it in about forty-five minutes." He predicts it will take the lifetimes of many more scientists around the world before anyone knows how to keep Jacesohn's Walden's heart beating in Ralph Sanduski without suppressing his immune system.

The secret of "selective tolerance," the ability of one being's tissue to accept another's, is deeply hidden in nature. If history is any indication, the quest to uncover it will come from breakthroughs in unrelated fields—like one that happened on a small farm in Scotland toward the end of the Second World War.

At a wound-treatment center near Glascow a zoology lecturer from Oxford named Peter Medawar was assigned to work with plastic surgeon Percy Gibson. After repeated failures of skin grafts made from healthy people to burn victims, Medawar hypothesized that rejection of the new tissue was an immunological event. He arrived at this theory after observing that the second attempt to graft skin from the same donor would reject must faster than the first. This, he deduced, was an example of immunologic memory, a phenomenon called "the second set response," which had been discovered in earlier studies on mice.

Having observed the rejection response in full force, the young Medawar could easily have accepted the conclusion of a prominent contemporary physician named Leo Loeb, who had audaciously pronounced a year or two earlier that "organizational differentials" in human beings would forever make organ and tissue transplantation impossible. It would never work, Loeb said. Fortunately, Medawar had also read of the work of a Danish scientist named Carl Jensen, who in 1903 had stumbled onto the fact that transplanted cancer tumors would be accepted by, and continue to grow in, genetically similar mice. Cells from the same tumors would be rejected by all other mice. Medawar also recalled the discovery of fellow Englishman Peter Gorer, who in 1916 confirmed that the genetic makeup of mice affected their tendency to reject or accept tumors. And there was the classic discovery at the University of Wisconsin that freemartin cows (a female born with a male twin) possessed a natural inborn blood chimerism (the existence of two blood types in the same animal). With these curious phenomena in mind, Medawar ignored Leo Loeb and continued his search for the mechanism that attacked foreign protein in higher life forms.

In 1948, while attempting with fellow British biologist Rupert Billingham to find ways to distinguish between identical and nonidentical (freemartin) twins in cattle, Medawar discovered to his surprise that freemartins as well as identical twins did not reject skin grafts from their siblings. Joined by Leslie Brent, a London-based immunologist, Medawar and Billingham began to reproduce the "freemartin" phenomenon in mice and discovered that when they injected tissue from one mouse into an unrelated newborn mouse, the second mouse would accept skin grafts from the first later in life. Here for the first time was proof that the immune response could be manipulated. Chimerism, two or more genetically separate tissues existing in the same organism, could actually be induced. It would seem possible, then, to transplant cellular tissue across histological barriers. Was Leo Loeb wrong? It was too early to know. Loeb had referred to humans, Medawar was working with mice and cows.

Medawar, Billingham, and Brent's work gave medicine its first rudimentary understanding of immunosuppression and convinced many surgeons that human organ transplantation could one day succeed. While it would be more than a decade before anyone found a way to control the human immune response, the foundation was laid with animal experiments. For his landmark discovery of "actively acquired tolerance of foreign cells," Sir Peter Medawar received a Nobel Prize in 1960. He died of a stroke in London on October 2, 1987.

HEALING

Following his transplant, Ralph Sanduski spent three and a half weeks in an isolated ward where everyone, including himself, wore masks to protect immunosuppressed patients from infection. As is the case with all transplant patients, Sanduski took a variety of drugs aimed at preventing his immune system from rejecting his new organ—Jacesohn Walden's heart.

"Everyone who came into my room looked the same," Sanduski remembers. "I even started to forget what Gretta looked like." By the end of March he was "feeling like a new man" and was tired of the Stanford hospital. On the twenty-ninth he was allowed to leave. It was a great occasion for the Sanduski family, all of whom were there to greet him. He would stay in the area for a few more weeks so that he could go in for regular chest X rays, biopsies, and blood tests. Compared to before, he was a free man.

That is not to suggest, however, that Sanduski will ever again live in good health. To combat rejection, his immune system will be compromised twenty-four hours a day, 365 days a year. If for only one day he forgets his little cocktail of olive oil and cyclosporine, followed by two steroid pills, he could die in a few hours. "The fact is, you have given up one disease for another," says fellow Stanford patient John L. LaBissioniere, who received his new heart in 1979 and is still experiencing the side effects of immunosuppression.

Norm Shumway has heard this before, and won't dispute it. "Transplantation involves a complete modification of life-style and permanent treatment with toxic drugs. There is definitely a downside." Shumway watches Sanduski and his other living survivors as closely as most people watch their children. The ongoing hazards of immunosuppression cause so much postoperative anxiety and depression among transplant patients that there are now psychiatric specialists who work only with transplant patients. Depression, anxiety about organ rejection, sexual impotence, unemployability, financial insecurity, and guilt about living because of someone else's death are the problems the new psychiatrists see in their patients.

"That's all there," says Sanduski, "but it beats the hell out of dying." He is back in Denver mowing that lawn, making love, and wrestling with his eight-year-old grandson. As "the shrinks" told him would probably happen, he worries some about rejection, death, money, and whether cyclosporine is damaging his kidneys. But mostly it's money, particularly when he looks at his $105,000 in medical bills, less than 80% of which will be covered even if he wins the fight he's been having with his insurance company. He wishes he had more sexual energy, wonders whether anyone will ever employ him again, and if Gretta is being too stoic for her own good. He thinks too, at times, about a sixteen-year-old boy whose name he will never know: "What would he be doing now if all this had never happened?"

REJECTION CONTROL

The Walden-Sanduski transplant was fairly typical. There were no extraordinary complications at either end. Walden at sixteen was a few years younger than the average donor, and Sanduski at fifty was about five years older than the average heart recipient. Within nine months of his operation, Sanduski had three minor rejection episodes, but all of them were detected by one of his monthly biopsies—early enough to alter his immunosuppressive regimen and stop them.

Heart biopsies are not fun. Each one involves a brief trip to a Denver hospital, where a "biotome" catheter with a small clipper on the end of it is placed into Sanduski's neck and worked down his jugular vein into his heart, where a small piece of myocardium is removed and brought back up the vein for analysis. There is no pain in the heart itself, because as it has been denervated; the nerves are not connected to the new heart. But the procedure is not something Ralph looks forward to.

Eventually, Shumway will find the optimal balance of cyclosporine A, azathioprine, and prednisome required to maintain Sanduski's heart and health. When he does, Sanduski will be able to reduce the frequency of his biopsies to one every quarter —but never to zero. Because his heart is denervated, it is impossible for him to feel the pain of angina, the major indicator of rejection.

No matter how frequently Sanduski's biopsies, Shumway will also watch his chart closely for the effects of the immunosuppressive drugs. Cyclosporine can cause kidney damage and high blood pressure, while side effects of the steroid (prednisone) he takes include osteoporosis, glucose intolerance, and, with some patients, psychological problems. He will return to Palo Alto at least once a year for a complete checkup. All his good luck could change in a moment, of course, but it seems he will be one of the patients whose outcome will improve Stanford's already impressive record which by the close of 1987 showed a 80% one-year survival rate, with 65% living two years, and 50% more than five years.

CHAPTER 6

LIVER

When handed a can of worms, I try to make butterflies.
PAUL TERASAKI, M.D.,
University of California, Los Angeles

About his specialty, University of Pittsburgh liver surgeon David Van Thiel says, "We hepatologists are ignorant about the liver, but we are becoming sophisticated in our ignorance." Much of the sophistication Thiel speaks of was brought to medicine by transplanters who, in the course of moving livers from one human to another, have learned many new things about this magnificent organ.

Weighing between three and four pounds, an adult liver holds a full 25% of the body's blood volume while at rest, though it will release a liter or so the moment it is needed for exertion. In a single day the liver will perform at least 500 vital metabolic functions, including the manufacture and release of more than a 1,000 different enzymes, the destruction of tired red blood cells (which are turned into bile, a combined waste product and digestive compound), the extraction of ammonia from amino acids, the conversion of ammonia into urea, the absorption of fat and its conversion to carbohydrate, the manufacture of blood proteins and coagulants, the processing of milk sugar (lactose) into glucose, the storage of lipid-soluble vitamins and proteins, and the detoxification of various poisons.

A sick liver is a serious and challenging medical problem.

Liver malfunctions are difficult to diagnose and are more often incurable than other organ failures. While many of the vital functions of kidneys, heart, pancreas and lesser glands have been mechanically or chemically replicated, few if any such duplications have been accomplished for the liver, though not for lack of trying. Even to perform the functions that *could* be duplicated artificially would require a chemical plant occupying several acres. And once the factory was built, there would still be hundreds of functions left that science has no idea how to perform.

JULIE

Julie Bornn has four years of high school ahead of her. While her friends in Yuma, Arizona, think mostly about the next four years, Julie tends to think more about the four after that. At fourteen, she is college-bound. She wants to study medicine at Johns Hopkins University, but if she is unable to obtain a scholarship there, she will settle for the University of Arizona 200 miles away in Phoenix.

Prior to March 3, 1987, Julie was by far the least likely of her friends to make it even to sophomore year in high school. She had a condition called Budd-Chiari syndrome, an obstruction of the hepatic vein, which caused her liver to swell to about three times it normal size. On January 16, 1987, the Phoenix-based hepatologist who had been treating her predicted that in less than a year her liver would give out. He referred her directly to John Brems, the brilliant young surgeon at the University of California, Los Angeles. It seemed like a long way to go to see a doctor, thought Robert and Sandra Bornn, until they arrived and found themselves in a waiting room filled with people from all over the world. UCLA hosts the largest liver transplant unit in the southwestern United States and every year examines hundreds of people with serious liver conditions.

The decision whether or when to transplant Julie Bornn was

no less complex than for any of the other serious liver cases John Brems had seen. Like so many of the diseases that ravage the liver, Budd-Chiari syndrome progresses slowly, and timing is vital. Transplantation is not always required. In fact, most often a Gortex shunt, inserted to bypass the hepatic vein, is a sufficient treatment for the syndrome.

One doesn't want to transplant an organ that might recover or be healed with simpler surgery or one that is still performing enough functions to allow a patient to carry on a fairly normal life, as was the case with Julie when she was first diagnosed. Nor is it good practice to wait until a patient is so sick that the surgery itself or even anesthesia might threaten his or her life. After Julie's first visit with Brems, he told her parents that it was a little early to decide one way or another. He took blood samples, ordered a liver biopsy, X-rayed her heart and lungs, performed an abdominal ultrasound, and released her to await results of the tests.

Not only would Brems and his colleagues in the liver transplant unit review the results of these tests, but they would ultimately take Julie's case before the UCLA Patient Selection Committee to determine her suitablility for transplantation. The committee is composed of surgeons, hepatologists, pulmonary experts, anesthesiologists, pediatricians, social workers, psychiatrists, blood bank personnel, transplant coordinators, and administrative officials. If the committee was convinced by Brems that Julie had an end-stage liver disease that could not be treated any other way, that she was psychologically stable and financially able to sustain a transplant, they would recommend it. It would take time just to get on the agenda of the committee, and more time to review her case.

"Can I go back to school?" she asked Brems.

"If you feel good, of course you can," he said.

The Bornns drove back to Yuma and Julie went back to school. For a few days she seemed to improve, until Sunday, February 8, when on the way home from church she fell asleep in the car. "Mom, Julie's asleep," said her eleven-year-old brother,

Jimmy. Sandra Bornn spun around and saw her daughter lying unconscious across the back seat, her skin a deep yellow. Had she slipped into a coma?

Robert Bornn drove as fast as he safely could to the Yuma hospital, where emergency physicians admitted Julie for diagnosis and treatment. Two days later she came out of the coma, but was unresponsive and complained of terrible headaches. Her upper abdomen was also badly swollen. The condition is called ascites and is characterized by an accumulation of fluids around the liver. It was obvious to all her physicians, including John Brems, who was consulting over the phone with her Arizona doctors, that she would have to be transplanted. Brems rushed her case to the Patient Selection Committee, which concurred. Julie's name was placed on the UCLA waiting list. That didn't mean that she would get a new liver, only that she would be in line for one her size from a donor with her blood type.

Brems called the Bornns and told them that Julie's chances of getting a new liver would be very much improved if she was in Los Angeles, close to the hospital. Yuma was simply too far away and too isolated to be certain that she would be there within the very short time (eight hours) that a liver remains viable after it is removed from a donor.

So in February of 1987 Julie and her mother moved to Los Angeles and rented an apartment about six blocks from the UCLA hospital. Like Ralph Sanduski, Sandra was given a beeper and told to stay close to a phone. She and Julie settled into a small but expensive studio apartment in Westwood, a trendy, upscale section of Los Angeles adjacent to the UCLA Medical Center.

Robert and Jimmy Bornn stayed in Yuma, Robert to run the store and Jimmy to attend school. Every day in the weeks that followed, Jimmy would come home from school; call his mother and sister in L.A.; talk about school, friends, and the swim team; watch a few cartoons while he did his homework; and throw a couple of frozen pot pies in the microwave in time for dinner with "Pop" over the six o'clock evening news.

Meanwhile in Los Angeles, life for Sandra and Julie Bornn

was lonely and boring. Even though Julie was able to remain out of the hospital and said she felt better than she had in the Phoenix hospital, she grew weaker and more yellow every day. And her stomach kept swelling. She never complained, except to say she missed her home and family. Sandra, normally an energetic and gregarious sort, began to brood. She would sit by herself on the bed and look at the floor while Julie watched television in the living room. She would become angry at the doctors for not finding a liver. Then she would feel sorry for herself. She felt guilty about her moods because Julie was so cheerful despite the weakness and headaches that seemed to get worse every day.

One day when she was taking Julie to UCLA for some tests, Sandra parked her car next to a Winnebago in the hospital parking lot. A woman about her age, standing next to the van, took one look at Julie and said, "Liver?"

"Yes," answered Sandra. "She needs a transplant."

"We're waiting too," said the other woman, who explained that her fifteen-year-old son, who was sleeping in the van, had been parked there for almost eight weeks. He too had Budd-Chiari syndrome.

Normally, Sandra would have been overcome with sympathy. This poor woman and her dying son would, in better days, have been recipients of her charity. She would have brought food, helped with cooking and cleaning, anything to make life easier for people like this. But all she could see at that instant was someone else in line for Julie's liver. She could barely speak or look the woman in the eye. Above all, she did not want to know her name or anything more about her son.

"We're late," she said as she took Julie by the hand and walked toward the hospital. As she rode up the elevator to Brem's office, she began to realize how the stress of caring for Julie had affected her. When she arrived at the transplant office, she asked for help and was introduced to Leslee Boyd, a social worker assigned permanently to the liver transplant ward.

Boyd was not at all surprised by Sandra's feelings. "The

wait is terrible, the very worst part of the whole ordeal, and it can last for months," she says. "People change a lot during those months." Boyd says she has to spend much more time with parents than she does with children. "Parents get angry that things are not going as smoothly as they thought they would. Some feel deep resentment when their child does not do as well as others. Others feel guilty if their child does a lot better than others around them."

Although tempted by the obvious advantage of their eighth-grade daughter being Yuma's first pediatric transplant, Robert and Sandra Bornn decided not to use the media. "I guess I had faith that the organ procurement people in L.A. would find a liver in time," says Sandra Bornn. "And I certainly did not want to be part of a 'Baby Jesse'-type campaign to move Julie ahead of children who had been waiting longer or needed a new liver worse than she did."

Financial as well as emotional stress can take a toll. Fortunately, the regional Blue Cross/Blue Shield carrier that covered employees at Bornn Hardware (a family business Robert inherited from his father) had recently decided to cover pediatric liver transplants (which they had previously considered "experimental"). Not all "the Blues" cover liver transplantation, but more are including it every year—most for pediatric cases only. Robert Bornn's earlier decision to pay the few extra pennies per employee per year to cover organ transplantation also proved fortunate.

But the Blues would cover only a portion of the hospitalization, which, the Bornns were told, could easily exceed $160,000 (the average cost of a liver transplant at UCLA). That meant that, in the best case, Robert Bornn would have to come up with about $30,000 for uncovered medical bills, as well as several thousand more for the apartment in L.A., not covered by insurance. All this did not include the $10,000 it would cost every year to keep Julie in the drugs she would need to combat organ rejection. Robert tried not to show his concern about money to Sandra and Julie, but he knew that no matter how it turned out, this illness meant the end of his nest egg. It was not until August that Sandra learned that Robert had liquidated his entire individual retirement account (IRA) just to cover preoperative expenses.

The fifth week in Los Angeles, Julie got worse. She began retaining more liquid and her abdomen swelled to about twice its normal size. It was a bad sign, Brems said. He admitted her into the hospital, where she continued to deteriorate. "She seemed so tired at times that she could barely open her eyes or speak," recalls Leslee Boyd. "Her behavior became bizarre. She became incoherent."

For the first time since they had moved to Los Angeles, Sandra Bornn began to feel the deep, terrifying fear that only comes when a child's life is threatened. She could barely make herself heard one late February morning when she called Robert and begged him to come to Los Angeles. "Please honey," she pleaded in a faint voice, "I need your help." Robert and Jimmy were there by her side that same day. The apartment was cramped with three of them, but Sandra was happier. She became more like her old self.

According to Leslee Boyd, tension often builds between the family of transplant patients and a hospital staff, particularly as the waiting patient's condition worsens. There were times when Robert and Sandra could barely see Julie through the forest of white coats clustered around her bed. It was especially disturbing to hear physicians disagree over how to interpret her symptoms. And some of the nurses seemed to resent the probing questions, particularly from Sandra: "Shouldn't she be turned over more often? Can't she have more than that to drink?" Brems calmly explained to her that liquid intake and sodium balance have to be carefully rationed and monitored in pretransplant patients. "If they get out of balance," he said, "it can cause serious complications during the operation."

About 10:30 on the night of March 2, about a week after Robert and Jimmy arrived, everyone was asleep in the apartment, except Sandra. The telephone rang. Before the first ring was finished, Sandra had the receiver on her ear and Robert had turned on the light. As she listened to the calm, matter-of-fact voice on the phone, Robert could barely recognize the expression that appeared on her face. For the first time in two months she was smiling.

"They have a liver for Julie."

MAKING BUTTERFLIES

Back in the late 1950s and early 1960s, a bold young surgeon-scientist at the University of Colorado named Thomas E. Starzl became determined to be the first man to transplant a human liver. Starzl, who had grown up in a small Iowa town, had already chosen the fledgling specialty of transplantation from the hundreds that had evolved in modern medicine (his second choice was oncology), and at Northwestern University and Colorado had established himself as a competent kidney man. But kidneys were too easy for this intense and notoriously impatient scientist. The actual kidney operation was fairly simple, and many others were fighting the battle against rejection.

Starzl could have chosen hearts, which were still untried in humans. But such individuals as Norm Shumway, David Hume, and Richard Lower were well advanced in their research. And again, the operation itself really didn't seem that challenging. But the liver was something else. There were more vessels to sew, agonizing and unpredictable complications, and everything had to move faster; there were no machines, as in a heart transplant, to perform the liver's function while it was out of the patient's body. Hemostasis (control of bleeding) is by itself more complex in a liver transplant than all the surgical procedures in an entire heart transplant.

It also appeared to Starzl—from early attempts with animals, at least—that the rejection response was more complex and enigmatic with the liver than with the heart or kidney. For one thing, he discovered that the liver seemed to be more immunologically privileged than other organs. Probably because of its size, it is able to absorb more antibodies than smaller grafts. And because the liver is overcompensated, it can lose a lot of cells and thereby suffer a great deal of immunological damage before the essential functions are affected.

Starzl, like a few of his contemporaries in the earlier days of transplant history, accepted the risk of bad publicity and the specter of legal action raised by transplanting animal organs into humans. Obtaining consent from patients' families to transplant baboon kidneys and livers into loved ones was never easy, but all of the human subjects of Starzl's early xenografts were terminal, so enough said "go" to keep the experiment alive.

In 1963 he performed his first human liver transplant. The patient died almost immediately, but it was a first, and firsts, whether successful or not, are badges of honor in experimental medicine. Four other patients were tried during the next seven months. They also died quickly. During the same time period, similar attempts were made in Boston and Paris, with similar results.

It was not until July 23, 1967, that Starzl performed the first "successful" liver transplant on a 1½-year-old girl. She survived for thirteen months. It was the same year as the world's first heart, pancreas, and lung transplants, and the same year that Starzl added antilymphocyte globulin (ALG) to the range of drugs that were being used to fight rejection. The age of transplantation had dawned and Starzl was there at the sunrise with heart transplanter Christiaan Barnard; Keith Reemtsma, the first to successfully implant animal organs in humans; Joseph Murray, who pioneered kidney transplants in Boston; and Jean Hamburger, the French nephrologist who became the philosopher-surgeon of European transplantation.

Tom Starzl is less acclaimed, however, for what may be an even more significant accomplishment than adding thirteen months to an infant's life—the combinating of azathioprine with prednisone, a formidable drug duet that worked noticeably better than either drug alone and remained the worldwide immunosuppressive regimen of choice until the advent of cyclosporine almost twelve years later, another transplant breakthrough in which Starzl played a significant role.

The growth, acceptance, and success of liver transplantation came more slowly than with other organs. Because the liver performs so many metabolic functions, there are just that many more things that can go wrong with a new one. For liver transplantation the operative mortality rate (meaning death on the table or within one month of surgery) was close to 40% in 1983. Today, the rejection rate has improved to around 30%—a troublesome figure, given the introduction of cyclosporine. And the longevity of liver recipients, an infrequently mentioned topic among transplanters, has never been that impressive.

Starzl will proudly point to a woman now living in South Korea, whom he transplanted seventeen years ago at the age of four, as the longest surviving liver transplant patient. But she is a remarkable exception to the rule. The one-year survival rate for liver transplants is about 70% nationwide. Five-year survival rates are less frequently published. Although claims vary widely from center to center, it is estimated that fewer than 40% of those patients transplanted experience graft survival after more than five years; of course, if they hadn't received a new liver shortly after rejection, they would have died. And according to Starzl, the twenty-seven patients that he attempted to retransplant prior to 1982 "bore bitter fruit." However, he said, "the few successes [in retransplantation] that have been achieved have served as an important stimulus for future trials." The University of Pittsburgh, where Starzl now practices, claims a 65% five-year survival rate for retransplants.

To be fair to all liver transplant statistics, one must keep in mind that transplant patients are selected from among the 50,000 Americans who die every year of liver failure. By the time they are transplanted, many are already perilously close to death, so their weakened constitutions hardly provide an ideal environment for successful transplantation. It must also be acknowledged that many of the early liver transplants that failed in the one- to five-year span were done in the pre-cyclosporine era, when less was known about how to control the immune response over the long term.

Starzl and his colleagues have had somewhat improved results with retransplantation, although the practice remains controversial in some circles and is, with the exception of pediatric transplants, still considered too experimental for most entitlement programs.

A more vexing problem facing transplanters has been their inability to figure out how to preserve a liver outside the human body for more than eight hours. The eight-hour "cold ischemic" envelope has placed enormous limits on their work. Only patients who are hospitalized or able to remain close to a transplant unit can be treated. Livers can only be moved long distances when there is standby private jet service available, and that is very expensive: most jet charters cost $1,000 to $1,500 for an hour of flying time. The short preservation time also prohibits HLA matching (tissue typing), which requires several hours of concentrated lab work.

Actually, transplanters disagree on the value of HLA matching for liver transplantation. Starzl says he has never seen a case of hyperaccute liver rejection (rejection immediately upon implantation), and postoperative testing suggests that tissue matching is not as important with livers as it is with kidneys and other organs. However, insufficient research has been done to determine the long-term effects of good and bad tissue matches on liver transplantation. Studies in animals do show that the mechanisms of rejection are the same with the liver as with other organs—they are simply slower. This may or may not be the case with humans. The best hope for improvement in liver preservation appears to be "UW-lactobionate," a new perfusion compound under investigation at the University of Wisconsin, where

Drs. Fred Belzer and Neville Jamieson have used it to keep dog livers viable for twenty-four hours.

TEAMWORK

While John Brems and his team flew south with Jacesohn's liver packed tightly in its picnic cooler, Sandra, Robert, and Jimmy Bornn dressed as fast as they could. As they walked the six blocks from the apartment to the hospital, the helicopter that shuttled Brems from the airport passed over their heads and landed on the roof.

Julie was anesthesized when Brems brought Jacesohn's liver into the operating room. Ron Busuttil, the chief liver surgeon at UCLA, had kept in constant radio contact with Brems and started the operation about thirty minutes before he estimated his partner would arrive. He did not remove Julie's own liver, although it was almost useless by then; even a weak liver is better able to provide some of the necessary metabolic and hemostatic balance than any machines or medicines available. Busuttil also had to be certain that Jacesohn's liver was healthy and would fit. A new liver can be a little smaller than the original and will grow to fill the space, but it cannot be larger than the original. There have been cases where, to save a patient, a liver that was too big has been sized down by removal or "resection" of a lobe. Surgeons have yet to achieve encouraging results with this procedure.

The Bornns waited in a nearby room especially set aside for families of patients whose surgery is expected to take many hours. They had been told they could be there anywhere from six to twenty-two hours depending on the number of complications that arose during Julie's operation. It was a large, comfortable room with long couches to sleep on, a television set in one corner, and enough magazines to keep anyone reading for a year. But Sandra Bornn could neither read nor watch TV. She stared out of the window at the jumble of buildings that make up the UCLA Medical Center. For a while she tried to imagine the worst, to prepare herself for the awful possibility of Julie's dying. "I don't know why I did that to myself," she told Leslee Boyd the next day. "I guess it was just something I had to put myself through—a sort of test of my ability to absorb the shock if it came."

For the first time, she began to wonder who it was who had to die so Julie could live. Could it have been as sweet a child? Was it a painful death? As the loneliness and terror became almost unbearable, she turned from the window and looked at Robert and Jimmy. She burst into tears and went over to them both. "I was so relieved that we were all together in one place," recalls Sandra. "For a strange moment it actually felt like Christmas." Then, without thinking what she was doing, she crossed the room and looked out a corner window that opened onto the parking lot. The Winnebago of the woman whose fifteen-year-old son needed a liver was still there.

Julie had been in the operating room for about two hours by then. The slow, meticulous removal of her sick liver had barely begun. Much had to be done before any of the veins, arteries, vessels, and ducts leading to and from the organ could be clamped, severed, and tied off. So much blood flows through the liver that even brief clamping of the hepatic artery, which carries oxygenated blood to the liver, and the portal vein, which brings it nutrients, causes a disruption of blood pressure throughout the entire body. So a bypass would be placed between the jugular vein in her neck and the femoral vein in her leg. The bypass would carry blood back from her lower extremities directly to her heart. Bypasses usually need to be placed only in adults, but Julie was tall for her age and Dr. Busuttil felt it should be done. Placing and later removing a bypass can easily add two hours to operating time.

The most difficult part of a liver transplant is removal of the patient's damaged liver. Life-threatening complications can arise with barely a moment's notice. Blood loss, for example, can be enormous. Sir Roy Calne, Britain's leading liver transplanter, shows a slide of him and his team standing in what appears to be about an inch and half of blood covering the entire floor of an operating room. "Things have improved since those days," says the witty supersurgeon, who is a popular speaker at medical conventions. What he means is that liver transplanters now have the technology to keep blood under better control. Most liver transplant units now include a "rapid infusion" machine that can replace lost blood as fast as it's needed. The UCLA version, with gallons of blood at the ready and manned by a special technician who never leaves his position at the machine, took up an entire corner of the operating room. Fortunately, it was not required in Julie's operation and the blood was returned to the local blood bank. The average blood replacement in a liver transplant operation is in excess of thirty pints per patient. Julie required only six.

The life-threatening possibilities of a liver transplant are so numerous that two anesthesiologists and sometimes an assistant anesthesiologist must be in the room at all times. There is a constant flow of nurses and technicians coming and going throughout the operation, most of them taking blood samples out for instant analysis. When blood is not being processed through the liver, its chemistry can change dramatically in a matter of minutes.

Unlike the talk during simpler surgeries, the dialogue in a liver transplant tends to be about the operation in progress. There is a steady stream of medical conversations, often two or more at once, one of them invariably involving an anesthesiologist who is being asked to recite one vital sign or another. A cryptic one-word command from Brems may set as many as four of the sixteen people in the room scrambling for instruments, sutures, sponges, and swabs. One nurse remains close to the operating room phone at all times to receive and transmit tests results from the blood lab in the next building.

"I'm almost ready for the liver," says Brems, by which he means he wants to begin sewing in the five or ten minutes it will take for a resident to check all the vessels leading to and from Jacesohn Walden's liver, making sure they are the right length and condition for the end-to-end joining of each vein, duct, and artery to their counterparts in Julie.

Now a lustrous oyster gray, Jacesohn's liver floats lifelessly in a stainless steel pan. In a strange way, it seems the only tranquil object in a room drenched in fluorescence, beeping monitors, stainless steel, and nervous surgical chatter. An hour of cautious stitching and tying, however, will restore it to the pulsating vibrant pink it has been a mere five hours before.

By now exhaustion is setting in, particularly among members of the team who traveled north for the harvest. Despite his own fatigue, Brems's hand is steady as he places the countless tiny stitches in the delicate vessels leading to and from the new liver.

It's hard to describe the mixture of excitement and relief that sweeps through an operating room when, after hours of detailed labor, clamps are removed from arteries and new blood flows into an organ—heart, kidney or liver; it doesn't seem to matter. That sudden surge of vitality somehow brings hope and energy to everyone in the room, no matter how tired they are. "It's what keeps us on our feet for twelve to twenty-four hours at a time," says veteran liver transplanter Nancy Ascher, who has done more than 130 transplants.

RECOVERY

Julie remained hospitalized for six weeks after her operation. About five days after the operation, she was released from Intensive Care, and Robert and Sandra took turns sleeping in a small cot placed next to her hospital bed.

To the liver unit staff, Julie's recovery was fairly routine. To the Bornns, it was an ordeal they will never forget, filled with uncertainties, whispered meetings, and more tension than they were prepared for. They soon learned that every increase in body temperature was a minor crisis, a possible sign of rejection. It was hard for them to accept that having a new liver did not mean that death had been defeated. The only thing that sustained them was Julie's indominable strength and contagious spirit.

Julie was released from the hospital on Good Friday, April 17, 1987. Brems asked that she and one parent remain in the area for another four to six weeks so that she could be carefully monitored on an outpatient basis. In a way, those were the hardest days of all. Sandra and Julie had already been away from home for three months, and Los Angeles with all its hassle and bustle was beginning to wear a little thin. The almost daily trips to the UCLA liver clinic were no fun either, with the endless waiting for appointments, drawing of blood, and probing of tender places. Finally, on May 19, Brems gave them the best news since that midnight call three months before. "You can go home now," was all he said.

According to Brems, Julie Bornn has done better than most of his patients. She has shown minimal signs of rejection, has plenty of energy, seems to be growing at a normal rate (a major problem for some pediatric patients), and is showing no side effects of cyclosporine or steroids. "She is even trying out for cheerleader," he says.

To Julie, things are not quite so rosy. Not long after she arrived home in Yuma, she began to get a bit puffy in the face, so slightly that even her best friends didn't notice, but Julie did and it bothered her a lot. The puffiness was caused by the steroid prednisone, which she had to take with her cyclosporine every day. She knew that, and grew to hate the drug and the very sight of the bottle it was in.

"Teenage culture is so obsessed with good looks, the slightest change becomes a major crisis," says Leslee Boyd. "Compliance is a particular problem with young girls like Julie. If they are not closely watched, they will independently cut back on their medicine. They will tell themselves that it is because they are feeling better, but it's really because they want to look better. And it works. If they lower they dose of prednisone, the puffiness usually subsides. They are, of course, playing with fire. And a lot of them don't believe it until they have rejected their liver."

Sandra Bornn watches carefully every morning while Julie

takes her medicine. It has become a time they both dread—Julie because she knows what it is doing to her face, and Sandra because she hates being "the wicked witch" who monitors her daughter's every move.

In October Julie was told she did not make the cheerleading team. The night she learned the news she didn't come down from her room to watch "Family Ties," a weekly TV ritual in the Bornn house. Fearing that she was depressed, Robert went to her room. The door was closed. He knocked and said, "Julie, aren't you coming down for 'Family Ties'?" There was silence. "Julie!"

"Dad," came the small voice through the door. "If I'm going to be a doctor, I am going to have to get A's in biology."

POSTOPERATIVE LIFE

Julie Bornn is unusual. She has done better than 95% of liver transplant patients. The postoperative course can be so much worse than the end-stage disease itself that the families have been known to pray for a merciful death for their loved ones—lying semiconscious, half-crazed by chemical imbalances in the brain, racked with pain and fever, and deeply depressed. Nurses and health workers often wish that liver transplantation had never been started in their hospitals.

Begin with the statistical probability that only 40% of the liver recipients alive today will live another five years. That means that six of the ten liver transplant patients who were released from UCLA the month Julie went home will not be alive in 1992. Before death, each will go through prolonged, agonizing struggles against rejection, infection, pain, ascites (fluid buildup), bleeding, pneumonia, and, of course, depression for everyone involved. The financial burden for some of these patients can quickly double or even triple the $160,000 the Bornns paid for Julie's transplant.

When they return to their hospitals, many of the patients will be approved for retransplant, at which point they will be placed on the top of the waiting list. This virtually automatic triage simply exacerbates the desperation, competitiveness, and resentment of those waiting for their first transplant. Retransplanting liver patients is, therefore, among the most hotly debated topics in surgical medicine. And the argument becomes particularly poignant in light of the fact that retransplanted patients have much lower survival rates than one-time transplants. "Why should someone with less of a chance of keeping a new liver get one before my child?" is the plaint of waiting families. And logically it is a good question, given the scarcity of livers, the high death rate among the waiting, and the decreased survival rate among retransplanted patients.

But working against these facts is an impulse stronger than logic, here described by Nancy Ascher, UCSF's recently arrived liver transplanter: "When you operate on a patient, you strengthen the contract you originally made with them and their family. It isn't something written or even spoken. It's something in your mind. I suppose it comes from our training. You just can't quit on them. You have to fight as hard as you can for someone you have operated on, no matter who else has to wait."

Ascher developed her skills at the University of Minnesota under the guidance of John Najarian, who says of retransplanting: "Once, maybe twice, but never would a Ronnie De Sillers happen in this hospital." De Sillers was a young boy who was transplanted four times at Pittsburgh before he finally died." Ascher supports her former boss on that policy but admits that if faced with a similar case, "I don't know . . . I just don't know what I would do."

When to quit on a patient is just something that no transplant surgeon wants to discuss. "Quitting violates the Hippocratic oath," says Ronnie De Sillers's surgeon, Tom Starzl. "Most surgeons I know would sooner quit their practice."

CHAPTER 7

BODY PARTS INC.

*Human beings have become useful to each other
in ways never before possible.*

EMMANUEL THORNE,
Aspen Institute

Eighty-three-year-old widow Adele Walker lives near a marsh on the northern coast of California. She is a passionate "birder." That's what bird-watchers call themselves in that part of the world. "I don't know much about birds," she confesses, "can only name a few. But I sure know the ones that settle here, how they behave and how they raise their young. Before my eyes fogged up on me, I used to waste whole days watching those little critters build their nests."

It was in 1984 that Walker's vision began to go. "For a while I thought my glasses were just fogged up. But when I cleaned them, I still couldn't see too clearly. After the lights dimmed, I didn't miss birding so much. After all, the birds were still there. I survived on sounds and memories. But after two springs of hearing all those sweet young chirps and reading about what was happening through a thick magnifying glass, I started to get depressed. I discovered that voyeurism was a powerful vice."

Walker reluctantly went to a doctor in San Francisco. He told her she had cataracts and gave her some medicine to slow down the fogging process. "This probably won't work," he predicted.

"You should be thinking about a corneal transplant." That sounded very serious to Walker. The doctor described it as a delicate but not very debilitating operation. "We just cut a thin circular piece from the clear outside layer on the front of your eye and replace it with a new one that we remove from the cornea of a clear-sighted donor." She said she would think it over.

Two more weeks without birds was all she could take. She called the eye clinic in San Francisco and asked to be placed on the waiting list. On March 4 the clinic called. "I collected my savings and headed to the city," she recalls.

Keratoplasty (corneal transplantation) was first developed by Austrian ophthalmologist Edward Zirm, who in 1905 took portions of cornea from a young boy who had died and placed them in the eyes of a workman who had been blinded by lime. The man's sight was restored until his death in 1908. It wasn't until the 1940s, though, that corneal transplantation was really perfected.

Although the instruments used in a corneal transplant must be extremely precise, the procedure itself is relatively simple. Under general anesthesia a small plug of cornea about the size of her iris was removed from Adele Walker's eye with a sharp circular cutting instrument called a trephine. The same trephine was then used to cut an identically sized plug from Jacesohn Walden's cornea, which had been stored for three days in a special tissue-culture medium prepared to preserve the extremely sensitive endothelium (layer of cells on the inside of the cornea). Taking great care never to touch the endothelium with any instrument or surface, Walker's surgeon carefully lifted Jacesohn's plug with a corneal spatula and inverted it like a tiny pancake into the hole that had been cut in Walker's eye. Working through a microscope, the surgeon then placed four "cardinal" sutures at 3, 6, 9, and 12 o'clock on the circumference of the graft, being careful to break only the outer surface of the cornea in order to preserve the delicate endothelium. Once the new plug was securely in place, a continuous circle of smaller sutures was made around the graft and tied off at the end with a tight single knot designed and placed to minimize abrasion of the eyelid. Once the circle was complete, the cardinal sutures were removed, and her eye was patched while the graft set.

Within a week Adele was back in her garden, "looking like long John Silver" with a patch on her left eye. A few days later she removed the patch. "I could see birds again. Only with one eye, of course. But that's enough for an old woman. I understand someone else needed the donor's other cornea."

That was an understatement. Almost 30,000 Americans like Adele Walker, from 3 to 103 years of age, blinded by injury, infection, inherited or congenital disease, regain their eyesight every year with corneal transplants. Had there been a sufficient supply of corneas last year, there could easily have been three times that number of replacements. When Walker received her new cornea, there were about 5,000 Americans in line for it. Jacesohn Walden gave sight to two of them. Archie Cochran, a sixty-two-year-old chemist who works for a West Coast coffee company, was the other. An expert in decaffeination technologies, Cochran was be able to return to work and retire with full pension at sixty-five. Although he paid almost $4,000 for his eyesight, Cochran considers his new cornea "a gift."

Jacesohn's corneas were not the last "gift" he left to humanity. After the surgical teams had harvested his heart, kidneys, and liver, and Nick Feduska had removed his corneas, three people from the Neuroskeletal Transplantation Laboratory (NTL) of San Jose came in and removed some bone, skin, and connective tissue.

For years the harvesting and storage of bone, ligaments, veins, nerves, cartilage, pericardium (the sac that encases the heart), mandibles, corneas, middle ears, skin, dura mater (the heavy membrane that covers the brain), fascia lata (a fibrous sheath that houses the major thigh muscle), and heart valves (if the entire heart isn't taken) have been a mere sideline of organ transplantation, mentioned in footnotes, if at all. But today, tissue banking has grown to become a vast and extremely competitive enterprise, one whose practices could reflect badly on the whole field of organ transplantation.

In 1986 more than 200,000 people in the United States received bone, tendon, ligament, and connective-tissue implants. The bone implants made up about half of the procedures. The cures and repairs made possible by these transplants are legion. For example, in addition to repatching the dura itself following brain surgery, dura mater is used for over twenty-five additional purposes, including hernia repairs, pericardium replacement, sheaths for peripheral nerves, spinal fusions, and the mending of cleft palates and lips. At surgical conventions anywhere in the Western world, one will find at least one booth in the exhibit hall purveying a brand of dura mater.

According to Shane De Vine, an official of the NTL, the next scandal that breaks in the transplant industry will be in tissue banking, although by all accounts it is unlikely to compare to the University of Pittsburgh's favoring of Saudi princesses over American patients—the 1985 case that created so much controversy for the transplant community. Gary Friedlaender, chief of orthopedic surgery at Yale University Medical School and former president of the American Association for Tissue Banks and of the American Council on Transplantation, says that "scandal" is probably too strong a word. Friedlaender is nonetheless extremely concerned about some of the trends he sees.

"The public is not aware that the tissue they are donating is passing through profit-making organizations before it reaches its destination," he says. "They will eventually discover it and the impact will be devastating—not only on tissue banking but on the whole transplant community." As aware as anyone else in the transplant community of the field's vulnerability to public disapproval, Friedlaender is "strongly opposed to any form of commercialization in organ or tissue procurement." During his tenure as president of the American Council on Transplantation,

Friedlaender led the fight against private organ merchants, who began trading in human organs before the 1984 Organ Transplant Act made that illegal.

Although most tissue bankers now abide by the letter of the law that makes it illegal to buy or sell tissues as well as organs, a lot of people, says Shane De Vine, are getting very rich in tissue banking. Although tissue is not, strictly speaking, bought or sold, he claims there is a lot of padding in the "processing fees" that tissue bankers charge with delivery of their products. It is a lucrative enterprise, and consumers appear to be paying much more than they need to for the final product. If there wasn't so much money to be made in tissue banking, it is hard to believe that the competition would be as fierce as it is.

Here's how it works. When there is a potential tissue donor in a hospital, morgue, or mortuary, a tissue banker will be called, probably by a transplant coordinator, and asked if he or she would care to harvest whatever the donor or his or her family has agreed to donate. At the appropriate time, technicians from the tissue bank arrive and take their tissues—bone, skin, dura, whatever. The tissue costs nothing, although a hospital might later bill the bank a few dollars to cover nursing or operating room time. Under no circumstances are any of the costs of harvesting organs or tissue ever passed back to a donor's family.

The technicians then take their harvest back to a laboratory where, in most instances, it is tested for viral infection, then sterilized; the donor is identified; and the material is packaged, frozen, and stored. When a surgeon or hospital orders a specific tissue, specifying size and shape, the bank delivers it with an invoice covering costs, which include the bill from the hospital and the tissue bank's own processing expenses, which are simply a calculated portion of bank overhead (salaries, rent, insurance, pension plans, public relations costs, and transportation). Ultimately, of course, these "processing fees" will be passed on to the end user, i.e., the patient who receives the transplant.

Processing fees for bone and tissues vary widely from bank to bank. Rib segments fetch about $150 apiece at the NTL. Bone dowels about an inch long cost $200, and a femur, or thighbone, might go for as high as $500. A whole knee joint is much more expensive at $2,600. Three small ear bones will fetch $750. Powdered bone is about $200 a gram at most banks (about four times the street value of cocaine). If the entire human skeleton were reduced to fine powder, it would be worth about $450,000, which begins to explain why so many people are getting into the tissue-banking business. In fact, the entire human skeleton is never harvested. But parts removed from a single cadaver can easily generate $25,000 in "processing fees" for a diversified tissue bank.

Tissue banking and transplantation have made the human cadaver, for the first time, an economically valuable item. Two decades ago the joke was that each of us was worth about $11.98—$10 for the gold in our teeth and $1.98 for the precious liquids. Today, most of us are worth much more dead than alive.

Friedlaender has no complaints with nonprofit tissue banks charging processing fees or even generating a profit from the proceeds—as long as the profit is being used to improve the infrastructure of the bank and the quality of the product. His complaint is with private, for-profit corporations and venture capitalists who have recently entered the field promising to pay dividends to passive investors. "I have no problem with free enterprise," asserts Friedlaender; "it just doesn't belong in tissue banking."

SUPPLY AND DEMAND

Like solid-organ transplanters, tissue transplanters are faced with an ongoing and chronic shortage of almost all tissues. In most instances, however, the demand/supply ratio is worse for tissues than it is for organs. "We probably don't come close to touching one percent of the need," says Bill Anderson, president of the Virginia Transplant Bank, of the situation in his five-state region.

Unlike organ procurement and delivery, tissue banking is a

virtually unregulated business. Because harvesting tissue is technically a rather simple operation, requiring very few credentialed or expert personnel, anyone with a few weeks' training and about $5,000 in seed capital can enter the field. The harvesting part of tissue banking, therefore, has many of the characteristics of a cottage industry. In fact, doctors have been known to take bone and tissue home and process it in their garages.

Wherever there is a large supply of cadavers one might find a tissue bank nearby. Small banks have even been set up inside hospitals, although most of them seem to have appeared in or near large tertiary-care hospitals where a lot of patients die and osteopathic surgeons create an internal demand for fresh tissue. It is often the surgeon, in fact, who starts and operates the bank. But most of the recent arrivals in tissue banking have been formed outside the hospital setting. Even a mortuary, the Lamb Funeral Home in Pasadena, California, created its own tissue-banking subsidiary called Coastal International Eye and Tissue Bank. The subsidiary ran successfully until the owners were investigated by local authorities for harvesting tissue without family permission, selling the product for profit, stealing gold teeth, and burning remains in a mass crematorium. Coastal International's departure from the business did little to alleviate the competition. In a densely populated area like Los Angeles County, it is not unusual to find as many as three tissue banks racing to harvest the same cadaver. Each of the banks will likely have paid a fee to separate staffers at the same hospital to tip them off when a donor becomes available.

The people who suffer most from this competition, of course, are the grieving families of people who have lost a loved one within the past twenty-four hours, usually a youngster, who, like Jacesohn Walden, died in a sudden accident. In the Los Angeles area a family might, in a single day, receive as many as three separate telephone calls from tissue banks, all of them "not-for-profit" organizations asking for donations. Until tissue banking is brought under regulatory control similar to that of the solid-organ procurement system, it seems unlikely that needless and self-destructive competition will subside.

The American Association for Tissue Banks (AATB) in Arlington, Virginia, has over 200 member banks and claims to be the self-regulating arm of the tissue-banking industry. But AATB executive director Jeanne Mowe says that many of the small "cottage industry" operations have not joined her organization and are therefore not bound to abide by its rigid code of medical standards. They are, in fact, regulated by no one. She says that counting those enterprises, tissue banks may number closer to 400 nationwide. She has no idea how much volume the industry handles.

THEM BONES

According to orthopoedic historians, bone has been successfully transplanted longer than any other body part, no doubt because, by itself, it is a noncellular material and therefore not as vulnerable to immunological rejection as an organ or cellular tissue like skin. Bone can be used whole to replace skeletal areas removed for cancer, severe trauma, or infection; small sections can be fashioned to strengthen or lengthen deformed spines and fill areas of crushed or fractured limbs; or it can be pulverized into a fine powder and used as a medium for dental and minor reconstructive surgery. In November of 1987 Dr. Richard Schmidt at the University of Pennsylvania in Philadelphia successfully transplanted the first whole knee joint into a bone cancer patient who would otherwise have had to have his leg amputated at mid-thigh. Similar operations have been done with elbows and shoulders.

Fresh autogenic bone (from the patient's own body) is, of course, the "gold standard" of bone transplantation. If everything is sterile and the transplant is done by the book, such a bone graft will take perfectly. However, allogeneic bone (from another donor, usually a cadaver) that has been cleaned of all cellular materials and either frozen or freeze-dried is giving autogenic tissue stiff competition. It was discovered almost accidentally that when bone was frozen before being implanted, the immune reaction to the graft was greatly reduced; and for reasons not yet clearly understood, that improvement seemed to work even better for freeze-dried than for deep-frozen tissue. But either way, this process has been found to result in a much stronger graft than metal or any of the synthetics that have been tried.

As it is a new and virtually unregulated industry, bone and tissue banking is rife with controversies and disagreements about how things should be done. Some tissue bankers, for example, feel that only bone and other connective tissue that are removed in a sterile (operating room) environment should be used for transplantation. Others feel that as long as the tissue is sterilized after removal and before it is frozen (secondary sterilization), it doesn't really matter whether the removal itself is performed in a sterile environment or in a merely "clean" one. Naturally, it is much less expensive to remove tissue in the latter. It can be done, for example, in a mortuary, at the morgue, or even in the basement of a hospital after an autopsy. And the "clean" operation can be performed far more rapidly than the sterile one, and by less skilled personnel. So it more likely to be the "cottage industry" firms that perform the "clean" retrievals, while the larger banks offer the sterile procedure. That fact alone may push most of the little guys out of the tissue-banking business.

Although there have been few reports of infections transferred to patients through donor tissue, two widely publicized cases in 1987 alarmed the tissue-banking community. In one, the patient died of Creutzfeldt-Jakob disease (CJD), a rare and fatal brain condition acquired in this case from a section of dura mater harvested in Germany. American tissue banks hastily claimed that Germany does not have rigid procurement standards. The other, reported in Britain, was a case of AIDS from a fresh skin graft. In the United States there have also been occasional reports of hepatitis, rabies, and CJD transmitted on corneas.

THE QUESTION OF PROFIT

Although most tissue banks are nonprofit and most of them are members of the AATB, some of the recent entrants in the field —which have either not joined or not been accepted by the AATB—are for-profit corporations. One such firm is Osteotech Corporation, a New Jersey–based creation of the New York City venture capital firm of Steinberg and Lyman. Steinberg and Lyman specializes in starting health industry–based companies with high-profit potential.

For the AATB and Gary Friedlaender, Osteotech is the most troubling new entrant in the tissue-banking field. When Steinberg and Lyman first launched the firm as a full-service bone bank in 1985, there was a strong and immediate reaction from members of the tissue-banking community. Quite simply, they resented seeing anyone openly making a profit in their field, although few if any of them were losing money. There was also some fear that a venture capital–driven corporation profiting from tissue *donated* by the survivors of dead people would bring bad publicity to them all.

Friedlaender and leaders of the AATB, arguing that tissue banks should be strictly nonprofit and administered by physicians, not capitalists, discouraged hospitals and medical schools from donating any bone to Osteotech. For a while it worked. Only two large hospitals—the University of Florida, whose chief osteopathic surgeon, William Enneking, was a founding director of Osteotech; and the Hospital for Joint Diseases in New York—agreed to send them bone. Others, including the Red Cross, refused to provide tissue to anyone profiting from its distribution.

Realizing that they would be unable to operate as a free-enterprise bone bank, Steinberg and Lyman hired Washington lawyer Steve Laughton, who formed a separate nonprofit (501-C-3) corporation called the Musculoskeletal Transplantation Foundation (MTF) to handle all the bone procurement for Osteotech. Osteotech, no longer in the procurement business (but still operating for profit), is today the fastest-growing state-of-the-art bone processor in the country. Since its formation, the MTF has signed up many more large hospitals and is actively negotiating with more. Osteotech's success, even its detractors admit, is due to the superiority of its product. "Nowhere can you get better bone," says Shane DeVine, himself a vocal critic of the Osteotech/MTF arrangement. "Yes, Osteotech is private and greedy," acknowledges Jean Mowe, executive director of the AATB, "and a lot of the industry is down on them. But their product is elegant."

Friedlaender, who does not disagree with Mowe or DeVine about the quality of Osteotech's bone, still insists that the MTF is merely a front for Osteotech and that their combined success in signing up medical schools results not so much from their superior product as from the financial support provided by the MTF to medical students and interns in the key institutions. He says it is nothing more or less than "payola."

VALVES

Another large private tissue bank is Cryolife Inc. of Marietta, Georgia, which calls itself "A Leader in Transplant Preservation." Cryolife, as its name implies, specializes in the cryopreservation (deep freezing) of aortic and pulmonary valves. Cryolife heart valves are later acquired by cardiological surgeons, who place them in patients whose own valves are worn, damaged, or deformed. In bold capital letters on the back of their six-page glossy brochure, Cryolife states, "We do not buy or sell human tissue or organs." In the strictest sense of the words "buy" and "sell," that is probably true.

The controversy surrounding Cryolife, similar to that involving Osteotech, has to do with the fact that the company is attempting to make a profit on the processing and provision (if not the sale) of body parts that were originally removed from hearts, which in most cases were donated for transplantation.

Often a donated heart is found unsuitable for transplantation. If the valves appear to be in good condition, the heart will be sent to Cryolife by either the hospital or the organ procurement agency (OPA) that retrieved it. Upon receipt of the heart, Cryolife will reimburse the sender for acquisition costs, which run about $450 for the average heart. Cryolife will then cryopreserve the valves and sell them to cardiologists and heart surgeons, who will in turn pass on their costs to the end user. A Cryolife aortic valve can be obtained for $2,995, a pulmonary valve for $2,595. That's a total revenue of over $5,500 from one $450 heart. Cryolife will not say how many hearts it strips down for valves every year, or how much profit there is in a single heart, but the enterprise supports about thirty-five well-paid employees and generates a profit.

The problem with the Cryolife system—and it is really no fault of Cryolife's—is that the donor family is often not informed that its loved one's valves may end up in a for-profit enterprise. This matter of informed consent should be the responsibility of the hospital, OPA, or surgeon making the original request. Cryolife claims that it informs its providers of the disposition of each valve and encourages them to inform donor families. Former transplant coordinator Amy Peele, however, says that by the time OPAs or transplant units are informed by Cryolife, a letter has already gone out to donor families, and most transplant coordinators do not want to send out another.

When Congress passed the Organ Transplant Act of 1984, it stipulated that no organ or tissue should be bought or sold. Otherwise, tissue banking was to be left unregulated. Sen. Albert Gore, Jr., sponsor of the bill, felt that since there was no federal money appropriated to tissue banks, they shouldn't be too tightly controlled. The allowance of "processing fees" was, according to Gore aide Jerold Mande, a concession to the industry. However, if the fee is unreasonable or it can be shown that the party procuring the tissue is profiting from it, then that party can be prosecuted under the act.

"It was also felt that adding tissue requests to the regulation would overburden the hospitals,'' explains Mande. ''It would mean that almost every grieving family would have to be asked for donation, not just the families of brain-dead patients.'' But some states that have passed required-request and routine-inquiry laws *do* include requests for tissue donations in their mandatory protocol.

LOOKING AHEAD

Whether human tissue is harvested from fetuses, brain-dead patients, or mortuary cadavers, its retrieval and distribution promise to be a hot item on the bioethical agenda for many years to come. Although less dramatic than organ transplants, tissue transplants will be much more widely practiced and affect many more people because the tissues from a single cadaver can go to many more recipients than organs from the same source. And because it is a very lucrative practice, the tissue bankers' defense of their enterprise, as well as their opposition to government regulation, promises to be vigorous.

PART THREE

BACKSTAGE

Sometimes it is insufficient to examine a technology by itself, it being merely a symptom of a larger paradigm. Such may be the case with organ transplanting, which is surfacing as the clearest metaphor we have for contemporary Western healing. Transplantation must be regarded, therefore, as more than a stand-alone technology. It should, in fact, be observed as a window on modern medicine.

CHAPTER 8

THE REQUEST

The donation of an organ for transplantation is probably the most exemplary gesture of human solidarity.

PROFESSOR JEAN DAUSSET,
Nobel Laureate,
Paris

Organ donation must be incorporated into the routine of critical care nursing.

PHYLLIS WEBER, R.N.,
Northern California Transplant Bank

Cadaver organ donation is, whether we like it or not, a family matter.

ARTHUR CAPLAN,
Bioethicist,
University of Minnesota

When Carol Fink asked Sam and Virginia Walden to donate Jacesohn's organs for transplantation, she had acted out a short and simple ritual with a long and complex history. She had learned the most recent version of the ritual only a month before Jacesohn was admitted to her hospital. By the time Jacesohn had entered

133

her caseload, she was comfortable with it. Though the seminar where she learned the new ritual did not delve into its history, the precise timing and careful wording of her appeal to the Waldens reflected three decades of legal struggle, ethical debate, and political maneuvering.

The step-by-step procedure for requesting an organ donation, though inspired by transplant surgeons who wished to legitimize the retrieval process, was actually designed in bioethical think tanks and refined in the private chambers of law and medicine. Today, the request procedure is proselytized and taught by transplant coordinators and organ procurement specialists who spend months of each working year "marketing" the needs and benefits of transplantation to the rest of the medical community and more recently in medical schools. Their objective is not only to raise people's awareness but also to alter the roles that intensive care nurses and other health workers play in the medical management of potential organ donors, particularly those hospital staffers who are reluctant to make the pitch for organ donation. "Medical marketing," a concept developed by Brandeis University sociologist Jeffrey Prottas, has taken the form of free professional education programs that often count for in-service training credit for the healthcare workers involved. The programs instruct intensive care and neurology ward nurses on the proper timing of a request and on methods of donor maintenance. Those healthcare specialties are deliberately targeted because 95% of all organ donors are declared dead in intensive care units.

The ritual of request is in some ways the most vulnerable aspect of the whole organ retrieval process. If it is not performed with great precision and sensitivity, there will be no organs. And without human organs, there will be no transplanting until surgeons have mastered xenografting (placing animal organs in humans).

Carol Fink was carefully instructed about the timing of her request. Here, from the *Journal of Neurosurgical Nursing* (April 1985) is the advice of Phyllis Weber, a registered nurse who became director of the Northern California Transplant Bank in San Francisco and an effective teacher of the ritual:

Timing: Only when the family accepts the finality of brain death can they be approached about donation. This timing is critical to obtaining consent; rarely can a family make a decision about organ donation without having time to reconcile their terrible loss. Notable failures in obtaining consent have come when the family has been asked for donation at the same time they were informed about the impending death.

When transplanters become too assertive in their pursuit of organs, they may confuse loved ones, alienate their peers in the medical community, and eventually scare the public. If they are not aggressive enough, however, they will harvest fewer organs. Some members of the medical community believe the transplanters are too aggressive. Most members of the transplant community believe they are not aggressive enough. The result is a subtle but persistent tension in and around most healthcare facilities where significant numbers of people are dying from brain injuries.

Amy Peele works hard to eliminate that tension. "It is a challenging undertaking to convince any healthcare professional that brain death is a sound diagnosis," says Peele, a former UCSF transplant coordinator. She designed a transplant liaison course there and taught Carol Fink the ritual in an intensive two-day seminar held in a downtown San Francisco hotel. "But once the staff accepts it comfortably, organ donation becomes a logical consideration."

A popular advisor to the American organ procurement community is Dr. Stuart J. Youngner of Case Western Reserve University in Cleveland, Ohio. "Staff should understand that human death and brain death are synonymous," Youngner writes in a widely disseminated paper entitled "Psychosocial and Ethical Implications of Organ Retrieval." "A brain-dead patient whose tissues and organs are merely functioning is essentially different from a living human being. . . . It is the life that remains in dead organ donors that makes their gift worthwhile.'' Hearing a doctor acknowledge that *life* remains in a ''beating-heart cadaver'' does little to reduce confusion among nurses and other ICU staffers.

Amy Peele's transplant liaison course teaches people like Carol Fink to carefully describe *all* the options faced by a family when a loved one dies of brain failure. The transplant coordinators at the University of California, San Francisco, have advised her to reveal enough detail so that relatives are able to give ''informed consent,'' but not to labor the specifics. She will never, for example, ask for specific organs at first. She will merely mention ''donation'' as an option, and emphasize that ''the gift of life'' can bring great solace in the future. ''This is one good that could come of your son's death,'' is the way one training manual recommends wording this particularly delicate part of the request.

''Don't be afraid to refer to the deceased by name,'' advises the University of California instructor at the two-day course, ''and avoid terms like 'cadaver,' 'corpse,' and 'remains.' Give the family time to decide . . . and remember that an initial 'no' sometimes represents denial of the death. It is not uncommon for a family to change their mind about donation after accepting the idea of death. So don't give up trying if they say no.

''Oh, yes, and don't forget to assure them that consent will in no way interfere with funeral plans—even with open-coffin viewing,'' counsels the UCSF instructor. ''Even if we take eyes, skin, and bone, the body will look natural in the coffin.''

Despite the dedicated efforts of Peele and her fellow transplant coordinators, some healthcare workers remain uncomfortable with organ procurement, particularly those who have to stay with the patient after he or she has been declared dead. ''It can be very depressing to care for a dead person only to retrieve their organs,'' said one nurse who asked not to be identified, ''especially a child.''

''I find it emotionally draining,'' said another. ''It is difficult to realize that you are taking all these extreme measures to preserve an organ, not a person. I have to continually remind myself that something good will come of this death.''

The most poignant sentiment was offered by a Chicago nurse who, when surveyed about her work with brain-death cadavers, said, ''I no longer think of them as people but as objects for salvaging parts—like a junkyard of cars.'' Peele, who has since left UCSF to become a transplant consultant, is troubled by that response. But she is patient, and confident that the time will come when health workers are more at ease with transplantation. ''Ideally, organ donation should be as unexceptional and as frequently undertaken as paying car insurance,'' Peele says.

Her efforts have borne fruit. A June 1986 position statement issued by the American Association of Critical-Care Nurses indicates that at least one professional organization has accepted her message. ''Organ shortage is not due to an inadequate supply of potential cadaver donors,'' the statement reads; ''it is due, instead, to the failure of healthcare professionals to identify potential donors and intitiate the organ donation process in a timely manner.''

SUITABLE VS. AVAILABLE

Transplanters believe that there is no shortage of *suitable* organs for transplantation, only a shortage of *available* organs. The ultimate goal for the transplant community is to make *all* suitable organs available.

Estimates of suitable donors vary widely from 2,000 to 60,000 cadavers a year, depending largely on what one considers ''suitable.'' The problem is that no conclusive studies have ever been made of potential supply, so all estimates are speculative. What is known is that between 1% and 2% of all the people who die in hospitals every year are legally and medically appropriate for organ donation. That suggests that 20,000 to 25,000 donors would be a more reasonable estimate. However, only about 3,000 of them are actually harvested in any given year. Transplanters, if they are to come even close to meeting the demand for their services, must find and harvest organs and tissue from the other 22,000. At that rate, there would be a surplus of most organs, and the most painful choice that transplant surgeons have to make —selecting recipients—would be eliminated.

To some degree, however, all estimates of supply must remain speculative as long as there are so many unforeseen factors affecting future supplies. Seat-belt, helmet, child-restraint, and speed-limit laws, for example, have an enormous and immediate impact on organ supply, as a majority of brain deaths in the U.S. (about 45%) still originate on the highways. When the federally mandated speed limit was raised from 55 to 65 mph, organ procurement specialists busily calculated that if all states implemented the new speed, as many as 9,000 more people would die on the highways and about 10% of them would become organ donors. That meant 1,800 more kidneys, 900 more hearts, 900 more livers, etc. Transplanters are cautious not to seem like lobbyists for highway carnage, but they do express their concerns. "The reduction in highway casualties has long been overdue," writes Dr. Felix Rapaport, editor of *Transplanation Proceedings*, a leading journal in the field. "It does, however, compel us to also re-examine the current sources of donor kidneys for transplantation purposes."

Handgun controls, of course, have had a negative impact on organ supplies. In some parts of the country, as many as 20% of brain-dead patients were once admitted to hospitals with gunshot wounds to the head. The improved proficiency of emergency trauma care has also had a negative effect on organ supply. San Francisco General Hospital's trauma center, where Jacesohn Walden died, for example, has an exceptional recovery record with head injuries. Transplant coordinators in the area, in fact, comment on the "disappointing" number of donors the hospital produces. "We only get about two calls a year from S.F. General," remarks Robert Capito at the Northern California Transplant Bank. Capito is, of course, glad that San Francisco General is able to save so many people, but he is concerned about the donor potential of some who don't survive. "SFG will fight for days to keep someone alive, and often those who could have been donors are worked on so long that their organs became useless."

And Capito is not alone with his lament on reluctant declarations and wasted donors. Donald Denny, former transplant coordinator at the University of Pittsburgh and considered by his peers to be the godfather of American transplant coordination, complains that "some doctors, even though they recognize brain death as diagnostic of human death, prefer to let a patient deteriorate on the ventilator until the heart runs down, as it inevitably will. That makes it extremely difficult on the family. They haven't been told their relative is dead. They have been told he is 'hopeless.' Their agony is prolonged." And the Pittsburgh transplant unit is out two kidneys, a heart, and a liver.

Transplanters are also painfully aware that one item of bad publicity or even a piece of fiction like *Coma* can affect the supply of organs immeasurably for years to come. *Coma*, a best-selling science fiction novel that was made into a popular movie, recounts the scheme of corrupt physicians who put patients into a permanent vegetative state and sell their comatose bodies to an organ farm called the Jefferson Institute. (At least every other person who knew I was writing a book about organ transplantation mentioned *Coma*. Some asked if I had found the *real* Jefferson Institute.) When the BBC in Britain aired a TV documentary called "Are the Donors Really Dead?" in which three people who had allegedly been declared brain-dead appeared on camera and discussed their experience, literally thousands of people tore up the organ donor cards they had previously signed. It was a grim day for organ procurement in Great Britain.

ORGAN MARKETEERS

Government schemes to allay the shortage of organs are as numerous and varied as estimates of their availability. One thing all solutions tend to have in common, nowadays, is their existence within the confines of the public sector. They are also based primarily on the process of asking for donation, i.e., the ritual of request. It wasn't always that way, however. Before passage of the 1984 Organ Transplant Act made it illegal to buy or sell human organs and tissues, free-enterprise visionaries offered their own solutions. "Will this emerging high-tech industry [transplantation] be run efficiently by dynamic entrepreneurs of the capitalist persuasion, or will it be semi-socialized and smothered by regulators?" asked a March 1984 editorial in *Fortune* magazine that railed against the Organ Transplant Act. The magazine called for an open market in organs that would provide real incentives to people who were "kidney rich and cash poor."

When cash-poor and kidney-rich Bob Reina of Ocala, Florida, placed an ad in the *Ocala Star-Banner* offering one of his kidneys for $20,000, he got no takers but was invited on ABC-TV's "Nightline," where he told his host, "You get to be thirty-five or forty years old and you see you've never accomplished anything, and you know you're never going to have five thousand dollars in the bank or any kind of security and you get kind of afraid. . . ." It was an appealing plea, reprinted by *Fortune* magazine in a second article favoring an open-market approach to organ sharing.

The *Fortune* articles were not well received by the transplant community. Though transplanters favored any plan to increase the supply of viable organs, they feared that an open market for them would shut down the donated supply. Some transplanters also had problems with the morality of buying and selling organs. "If you say a person has a right to sell off a bit of himself if he wishes and you argue that to its logical end," said Oxford University's Dr. Peter Morris, past president of the International Transplant Society, "then you arrive at the same point as the prosuicide groups. Selling yourself is not an individual action. It demeans society as a whole. In fact, it creates two societies in which the poor grow organs and the rich reap them."

The controversy was a rich lode for American bioethicists, particularly an emerging subgroup among them who were finding transplantation an attractive specialty. Arthur Caplan, the unheralded dean of transplant ethicists, is now a professor at the University of Minnesota, which houses the country's second largest transplant unit. He believes that "while there may exist those who are desperate enough to sell all or parts of their body for money, it is surely not in their best interest to allow them, much less to encourage them, to do so. Surely our society can find better ways to solve the problems of poverty than permitting people to sell vital organs, or families to parcel out the bodily remains of their loved ones, to the highest bidder."

Caplan's remarks invoke visions of an organ exchange with daily price quotations, a futures market, and organ brokers working on commission. One can also imagine kidneys being offered as collateral for personal loans, the application for which would include organs as a measurement of net worth. As farfetched as that seems, Dr. H. Barry Jacobs of Reston, Virginia, actually attemped to create an organ brokerage company as recently as 1983. Jacobs made no effort to hide his motives or his values. This could be "a very lucrative business," he told a Virginia newspaper. "If the 'haves' want it, they will have to pay; if the 'have-nots' want it, they will have to pay too." The scheme, opposed by almost everyone else in medicine, all the way up to and including U.S. Surgeon General C. Everett Koop, was stopped by Virginia authorities, not because the idea was necessarily a bad one, in their estimation, but because Jacobs was a convicted felon. Georgetown University medical ethicist Robert Veatch objected to Jacobs's idea on historical and practical grounds. If the organ market turns out like the blood bank economy, he says, the quality of organs will decline drastically. "People will have an incentive to hide potential problems—a history of kidney disease, a disease in the family, or possibly even a terminal illness."

A slightly more respectable scheme was floated in 1985 by

William von Meister, the millionaire computer tycoon who designed Western Union's electronic mail service and The Source, a successful computer data bank. Von Meister, aware of the recently legislated restrictions against buying or selling organs, instead proposed a $15-a-year insurance plan that would guarantee a suitable organ to the policyholder. Von Meister intended to acquire his organs by offering to make a $10,000 donation to the charity of the donor's choice. He received predictable opposition from the transplant community: Oscar Salvatierra, Jr., president of the American Society of Transplant Surgeons, called the idea "immoral and intolerable." Von Meister was able to garner more support for his plan than Barry Jacobs could for his. Baird Helfrich, for example, the prominent kidney surgeon from Georgetown University Medical Center who performed a top-secret transplant for Ferdinand Marcos, agreed to sit on von Meister's board of trustees (as "medical adviser" to the plan), a decision that did little to advance Helfrich's respect or popularity in the transplant community.

When confronted with his support of the plan, Helfrich admitted that von Meister was "off track, but not evil. He's just a capitalist practicing the good old American business of making money," he told the *Pittsburgh Press*. If it was shown to be "a profitmaking activity," however, Helfrich promised to "withdraw from the board."

Milton Friedman, the high priest of untrammeled free enterprise, has reservations about buying and selling organs. Recalling eighteenth-century grave robbers who exhumed the dead to sell cadavers to medical schools, Friedman fears that "if the price is right, some might be moved to kill people for their organs." *Fortune*, which normally adulates Milton Friedman, remains unimpressed. "There is precedent for opposition to certain markets," an article reads; "prostitution and the sale of babies come to mind—but with organs the consequences of shortage are tragic." The implication is that an open market would increase the supply of organs, a conclusion that few transplanters would support.

Judging by the overwhelming congressional majority that passed the Organ Transplant Act, there seems to be little agreement with *Fortune*'s position of this subject. Free-enterprise medicine is generally considered inappropriate for organ transplants. For example, if the marketplace is allowed to rule, it seems likely that transplants would become a service for the few who could afford to buy organs from those desperate enough to sell them. The "living will" would become a living sales slip and families of brain-death victims could become waiting-room auctioneers to families of the dying. Capitalism would mar the noble act of giving the gift of life. Donald Denny, at the University of Pittsburgh, sounds a warning: "Should the American public's support of [voluntary] organ donation ever falter, transplantation in this country would come to a halt. If abuses of the system are not stopped immediately, the damage to the trust we have worked so hard to build will be irreparable." In his view, organs-for-profit could undermine public support; thankfully, Denny and people who share his opinions have prevailed. Richard Fine, chief of clinical services at San Francisco General Hospital, is relieved. "One of the greatest victories in modern medicine," he says, "was the defeat of the private organ merchants."

ANATOMIC GIFTS

Defeating the organ profiteers did not, of course, solve the supply problem. Despite an innate disdain for regulation, the transplant community began in the late 1960s to explore legislative solutions to organ shortage. Having a few supportive health workers willing to make the request—whether to an individual, a family, or an entire nation—was clearly not sufficient. Furthermore, the legality of request, donation, and recovery of organs was clouded. Clarity could only be brought with legislation, transplanters w beginning to realize.

Prior to 1968, which became a pivotal year in tr

history, most state laws concerning disposition of the dead were confusing. When surgeons first began transplanting humans in the early 1960s, the recovery of organs from cadavers was loosely covered under common law provisions affecting the use of unclaimed cadavers for research. But some states required such cumbersome legal rituals before an organ could be removed that surgeons could transplant only "out-of-state" organs—those harvested in a neighboring state and transported across the border.

Any delaying factor is an obstacle to transplantation, which requires fresh organs swiftly removed from respirated (beating-heart) cadavers. As legal problems mounted for the transplant community, and the demand for healthy organs escalated, the National Conference of Commissioners on Uniform State Laws (NCCUSL) was asked by an ad hoc committee of surgeons and physicians to draft a model organ donation bill. It was an awesome political challenge to draft a law acceptable to fifty separate state legislatures in a nation where individualism and individual rights are prized, where so many religious faiths flourish, and where there remained much legal and traditional confusion about who had the right to determine the fate of the dead or, more important, who owned their organs.

However, the NCCUSL rose to the challenge. The result was the Uniform Anatomical Gift Act (UAGA), which was sent in draft form to all fifty legislatures in July of 1968. In summary, the proposed bill provided that:

1. Anyone over 18 may will or donate all or part of his or her body for science or transplantation.
2. If the individual has not willed his or her body before death, his or her relatives may donate it.
3. If there is more than one relative with the same degree of kinship and one is opposed to donation, he or she prevail.
4. No willed donation may be revoked by relatives.
5. The donation can be authorized by a card carried by the donor or by written or recorded verbal communication to a relative.

6. The donation can be revoked at any time before the death of the donor.
7. The time of death must be determined by a physician not involved in transplantation.
8. Organs may be donated to a hospital or a surgeon, for research, to an accredited medical school, to an organ bank or storage facility, or to a specific individual.

By 1972 some form of the UAGA had become law in every state and the District of Columbia. It was the fastest-known enactment of uniform legislation in American history. The act deliberately omitted a definition of death, a provision considered so controversial that the act would never pass if it were included. The medical community was probably right, but as we shall see, that didn't stop them from later proposing separate legislation that redefined death, in part for the convenience of organ transplanters.

After passage of the UAGA, anyone anywhere in the United States carrying an organ donor card in his or her wallet who died of brain injuries in a hospital was a potential organ donor. Doctors could (and still can) legally harvest organs from a card-carrying donor without asking permission of relatives. In fact, in the U.S., that rarely if ever happens. The sanctity of family and medical tradition, which regards the living as more important (and powerful) than the dead, still prompts doctors and hospitals to ask the next of kin for permission to harvest organs. Like San Francisco General, all large hospitals now have elaborate protocols for soliciting organ donation, most of which mandate an aggressive twenty-four-hour search for family members that must be carried out before organs can be removed. If a spouse, parent, or sibling of a patient is found and says no, the hospital will abide by the family's request, even if the patient carries a signed donor card.

The problem with the UAGA was that it assumed, perhaps naively, that healthy people would contemplate their mortality, make a conscious decision to allow the surgical removal of their organs after death, and sign a document permitting it. This premise flies in the face of our most basic understandings of mortality, perhaps best articulated by Sigmund Freud, who said:

Our own death is indeed unimaginable, and whenever we make some attempt to imagine it, we perceive that we are really surviving as spectators. Hence, at the bottom, no one believes in his own death, or to put the same thing another way, in the unconcious everyone is convinced of his own immortality.

Veteran Stanford University heart transplanter Norman Shumway has a simpler theory: "I think a lot of people think to themselves, 'If I sign this donor card, I'm going to die.' "

One empirical proof of the Freud and Shumway theories is that very few people have ever signed their donor cards. Despite polls that consistently show that about half of all Americans are willing to donate their own organs, less than 20% actually sign cards and only about 5% carry them—even in states with vigorous publicity campaigns and cards printed right on the back of driver's licenses. (In Colorado, where drivers are *required* to check off 'yes' or 'no' before they are issued a license, about 60% check the 'yes' box. But Colorado is the only state with such a requirement, and physicians will still abide by wishes of a family and ignore the card.)

In a way, it is irrelevant how many people have signed cards. As a general rule, even people who have signed them don't tend to arrive in an emergency room with the cards on their person. The real value of the organ donor card is as a consciousness-raising device. A single card can stimulate a family to discuss organ donation. Transplant coodinators report that families who have discussed it are generally willing to abide by their loved ones' wishes and donate without hesitation.

Although there can be no doubt that by the mid-1970s the UAGA and donor cards had improved the supply of organs, they came nowhere near meeting the demand. Something more had to be done.

STATUTORY REQUEST

Why not float another bill, some transplanters asked, one that would require all hospitals to approach the families of brain-death patients whose organs were still intact and suitable for transplantation? The idea was first proposed by Hastings Center bioethicist Arthur Caplan, a jovial, fast-talking intellectual who by 1984 was seen as a fairly good friend of the transplant community. Hastings, which Caplan left in 1987, is a think tank north of New York City that has become a major center for bioethical research and consulting. Bioethical consulting has itself become a small growth industry in modern medicine. Hastings has 11,000 paying members, but is funded primarily by foundations and corporations, including the Sandoz Chemical Company, makers of cyclosporine A, the most widely used immunosuppressive drug in transplanting.

In a Hastings Center *Bulletin* dated October 5, 1984, Caplan proposed an organ procurement strategy he called "required request." "Our society's decision in the late 1960s to rely on a public policy of voluntarism as the primary means of assuring an adequate supply of organs for transplantation is no longer tenable," Caplan wrote. Legislation should be introduced at the state level, he said, *requiring all hospitals to request organs and tissues from the survivors of brain-dead patients*. Any hospital refusing to make the request should lose state Medicare reimbursements. To Caplan, required request was a compromise between more authoritarian European practices of "presumed consent," or "implied consent," and nothing. It was also, Caplan argued, a way of preventing an open market for cadaver organs.

Ideas like Caplan's request proposal tend to remain submerged for a few years. Surgeons and physicians, like any professionals, typically keep their controversies to themselves, at least until they are close to agreement or compromise. So for months required request was discussed quietly, in unscheduled meetings at medical conventions, over the phone, over drinks, over breakfast, but never before the public or the press—at least not until it was agreed that a palatable version and an inoffensive strategy had been found. It was, after all, a fairly authoritarian proposal.

While discussions were under way in the inner sanctum of medicine, a human drama was playing itself out in Oregon that would make Arthur Caplan's proposal more appealing to the legislators in that state. Back in October of 1982 a baby girl named Denita Alexander had been born with biliary atresia, a congenital blockage of the bile duct that can be remedied only by a liver transplant. Her unwed mother had given her up to a foster mother named Mary McDermott, who immediately began the long and painful search for a transplant unit that would take Denita. When the University of California, Davis, agreed to accept her as a patient, state Medicaid officials in Orgeon refused to cover the operation. It was "too experimental," they said. McDermott went to the media and together they publicized the case. After a two-year battle with bureaucrats and legislators, a special exception was made for Denita and the state of Orgeon agreed to cover her transplant.

Denita, by then two and a half years old and weighing only eighteen pounds, had become Oregon's first transplant media darling. The whole state followed her ordeal as Mary McDermott hunted desperately for the scarcest of all commodities—a liver that would fit in the tiny emaciated body of a dying girl. In March of 1985, with Denita in critical condition, a liver was found and transplanted. Eleven days later it failed. Another was found, but it, too, failed and Denita died.

Larry Hill, a state congressman from Denita's district who watched the drama unfold and happened to have read Caplan's proposal, thought it a propitious time to introduce required-request legislation in Orgeon. However, when Caplan had drafted his original proposal in the ivory towers of Hastings-on-Hudson, he failed to take into account the power of semantics. "Required" is a word loaded with authority, certain to raise the ire of doctors, hospital administrators, and the national organizations formed to protect their respective interests. Indeed the Hill bill was vigorously opposed by health workers who resented having to approach grieving families and ask for loved ones' organs. It also alarmed the public, which had by then grown a little suspicious of the transplanters' relentless pursuit of organs.

"That's where I learned my first lesson in semantics," admits Caplan in his new office at the University of Minnesota. "I changed my proposal to 'routine inquiry' and got much less resistance." "Routine inquiry" was subtly, but importantly, different from "required request." The latter would force hospitals to *ask* for organs. Routine inquiry simply mandated them to adopt a protocol whereby the survivors of brain-dead patients would be *advised of their options*. One option advised, of course, would be to donate organs.

On June 7, 1985, Oregon passed the nation's first routine-inquiry law. Dubbed by the media "Denita's bill," it was signed into law a month later. The idea caught on fast. Similar bills were introduced and debated in most other states of the nation. In the first six months of 1986, fifteen states passed either required-request or routine-inquiry statutes. By mid-1987 forty-two other states had request laws, and routine inquiry was the spirit of a federal regulation mandating all federally funded hospitals to adopt an organ procurement protocol. That rule went into effect on October 1, 1987.

It was the routine-inquiry law of California that Carol Fink was acting under when she approached Sam and Virginia Walden, which is why she didn't actually ask for Jacesohn's organs. She simply told the family they had the option to donate them. Fink says she likes having the law behind her. "When I am uncomfortable making the request or anticipate a negative response," she simply tells the family of the deceased, "The law of the state requires me to inform you of your option to donate organs."

Some states, like New York, managed to pass more strongly worded statutes—closer to Caplan's original required-request proposal. So far, however, there is no evidence that more aggressive statutes produce more organs than the gentler routine-inquiry laws. There is also little evidence to indicate, one way or another, whether required-request and routine-inquiry laws are responsible for the gradual increase the transplant community has experienced in organ retrieval. The laws have opened hospital doors to organ procurement agencies who not only offer their free educational programs but also make frequent "social calls" to ICU nurses and staff. It is too early to assess the impact of that phenomenon on intensive care and grief counseling.

Some transplant surgeons with long waiting lists who regard the organ shortage as a "national public health crisis" are calling for even stronger statutes. Some even propose laws based on the European concept of "presumed consent," also referred to as "implied consent."

STATE PROPERTY

Following an example set by France, Israel, Greece, Norway, Italy, Switzerland, Finland, Sweden, and Denmark passed laws mandating the right of a hospital or transplant surgeon to remove organs from the body of anyone who hasn't written a will or declaration to the contrary. Under presumed-consent, or implied-consent, laws, instead of voluntarily "opting in" to organ donation, people have to actively "opt out" or their organs can be harvested without anyone's permission. Poland, Czechoslovakia, and Austria have passed even more authoritarian statutes which say that organs, at the moment of death, become the property of the state.

It is interesting to note that in six of the countries that have passed presumed-consent laws (Finland, Greece, Italy, Norway, Spain, and Sweden), some doctors and hospitals still make every effort to find the next of kin, and act on their wishes, even though they no longer need to. If they can't find the family, of course, they will most often go ahead and take the organs. Transplant surgeons interviewed in France in the spring of 1987 varied widely on presumed consent, some saying that they would never take an organ without permission of relatives, others that they would never bother to ask.

American transplant surgeons are, by and large, strongly opposed to presumed-consent bills. They reacted vociferously when Arthur Caplan floated the idea in 1983. Although they admit that such laws might produce more organs for a while, they fear that the healthy American aversion to state authority would eventually result in a reaction that could, in the end, lower supply. The very same 70% of the population that, according to polls, now "opts in" to organ donation might very well "opt out" if *forced* to chose between a presumed "yes" and a declared "no."

Outspoken opponents of presumed consent like Oscar Salvatierra, Chief transplant surgeon at the University of California, San Francisco, and former president of the American Society of Transplant Surgeons, say that the French practice of asking for donation, even though it's not required, simply "proves that presumed consent won't work."

Thomas Starzl, chief of transplant surgery at the University of Pittsburgh, the world's largest transplant unit, is not convinced by Salvatierra's logic. In an editorial published by the *Journal of the American Medical Association* on March 23, 1984, he wrote, "Implied consent has never been used in the United States, but this may represent only the past prejudices of physicians rather that the future prospects of this approach. The ease and uniformity with which cadaveric organ donation under conditions of brain death was accepted by society came as a great surprise two decades ago to transplant surgeons who did not appreciate the wisdom and altruism of the public at large."

Starzl, one of the most controversial surgeons in the field, knows the risk he takes by promoting "presumed consent" in America. But he is philosophical about it. "I think if someone wants to enter the political arena and all that that entails," he told a recent gathering of bioethicists in Boston, "including getting shot at by every nut that passes by, you might as well do it for something worthwhile, which is to ask for what you need, which is presumed-consent laws.''

Robert Veatch, bioethicist at Georgetown University and strong advocate of organ transplantation, counters Starzl's logic. ''Any scheme,'' he says, ''that abandons the mode of donation in favor of viewing the cadaver as a social resource to be mined for worthwhile social purpose will directly violate the central tenets of Christian thought and create some problems for Jews as well.'' It is unlikely that such legislation will soon pass in the United States. It seems too soon to give up on voluntarism.

Veatch, however, proposes a considerably different model of required-request law than any of those in existence. Similar to the Colorado driver's-license law, Veatch believes that ''while we are healthy and competent, we should all be required to answer the question of whether or not we are prepared to donate our organs.'' He calls it ''compulsory question answering.'' Instead of using the driver's license as a medium for approval, Veatch prefers either the tax return or the standard questionnaire handed to anyone entering a clinic or hospital for any reason at all. ''We are already asked fairly personal questions on our tax returns, like whether we will designate part of our taxes to a particular political party. Under compulsory question answering we would be asked routinely, on an annual basis perhaps, whether we are prepared to make a donation. The updated information would be stored on centralized computers accessible to transplant teams.''

Veatch's proposal appeals to Leo J. P. Clark, a Toledo, Ohio, neurosurgeon who spends a good deal of his spare time crusading against organ procurement—''not organ *donation*,'' Clark is quick to point out, ''organ *procurement*.'' Clark, a bête noire of organ transplanters, whose name is openly reviled at transplant conferences, has appeared frequently before state legislative committees considering required-request statutes. ''There is a growing political force in this country,'' he wrote to a state senator in 1986, ''which holds that the rights of some individuals in our society to obtain organs are greater than the rights of other citizens to privacy and medical consent during a period of emotional turmoil in their family.

"It is my observation," Clark continued, "over ten years of practice, that most 'organ donations' are actually organ procurements obtained by the coercion of family members who are in a state of emotional shock and very vulnerable to manipulation. Imagine the scenario of a family huddled in prayer outside an intensive care unit, hoping against hope that their twenty-year-old daughter will survive a serious head injury. Typically in this setting, guilty feelings arise over whether this accident could have been foreseen or prevented. . . . Enter an authority figure dressed in white, perceived by the family to be knowledgeable about matters of medical care, who interrupts their anguished prayers to say, 'Mrs. Jones, your daughter's not doing very well and I was just wondering, have you given any thought to donating her organs?'

"The suggestion that they *should* be thinking about donating her organs is an absurdity. Of course they're not thinking about organ donation. They are thinking about the wedding they were hoping to attend next June. They are thinking about all those Christmas mornings, the day their daughter left for college, all the things they wanted to say and may never get to say. They are thinking of their mental pain and anguish in this the darkest hour of their lives.

"Were they of sound mind, they would ask 'Mr. Dogood' to mind his own business and possibly ask him who the hell he thought he was, invading their privacy with such a question. Unfortunately, most families have frequently been up all night with no sleep, are emotionally and physically exhausted and easily manipulated. The suggestion by an authority figure that they should be thinking about organ donation often increases the sense of guilt that they were not.

"To create a law that every family anguishing near the ICU be confronted regarding organ donation is, to my point of view, highly inappropriate."

Leo Clark's point of view has clearly not prevailed. It has

been effectively countered by the persuasions of the transplant lobby. "It is hard for people in my profession [neurosurgery] to embrace my position, particularly in large institutions," says Clark. "The same patient whose intensive care for trauma injuries might cost a hospital $250,000 could also provide the raw materials for $2 million worth of transplant surgery. If a neurosurgeon at the University of Pittsburgh said what I am saying, he would be out of a job."

At Montefiore Medical Center in New York City, a physician with Clark's attitude might not be out of a job, but he or she would certainly have words with kidney transplant surgeon Dr. Vivian Tellis. Tellis, whose seventeen-year-old brother died on a respirator, has problems with people who refuse to donate organs. "Instead of feeling good and righteous about donating," he asserts, "it should enter the collective unconscious that we feel bad if we refuse. People who refuse should be informed of the consequences." Tellis explains: "Before a family finally refuses consent, they should be made aware that people are dying for need of these organs and that as a consequence of their saying no, there will be somebody who will be badly served by it.

"But they should never be told that they had killed a waiting recipient," he adds. "*That* would be going too far."

PERSISTENT SCARCITY

Although the public has largely come to accept the idea of transplanting and, to a lesser degree, donating organs, promotion and professional education do not appear to have completed the job. As sociologist Jeffrey Prottas, a strong proponent of "medical marketing" by the transplant community puts it: "Altruism is not easy to sell, [even when] all major religions and the generality of public opinion consider it a 'prestige product.'" Scarcity still persists, as waiting lists at major transplant centers attest. Dying patients and impatient families challenge weary surgeons to make miracles, and healthcare workers, like Carol Fink, who were trained to counsel the grieving, are retrained to watch also for potential donors, and when they see them, to ask for their organs.

The shortage, particularly of hearts, will not be allayed in the foreseeable future. In 1986 it was estimated that between 14,000 and 15,000 people die in the U.S. every year who could have been saved by heart transplants. Another 15,000 nonterminal heart patients could have benefited greatly from transplants. Yet even with optimal procurement, there would have been only around 1,500 viable donor hearts harvested during the same time period. A similar, though not as extreme, imbalance exists with livers, and it will almost certainly exist for pancreases when pancreas transplantation is perfected and a million insulin-dependent diabetics become potential recipients. These ratios help to explain the boldness of transplant coordinators, the competition among hospitals and organ procurement agencies, the intense research efforts under way to develop artificial organs, and the willingness of at least one surgeon to experiment with baboon hearts in dying human babies. And it all adds an urgency to the ritual of request.

As transplanters advance their techniques, survival rates lengthen, and the quality of postoperative life improves, it seems certain that more government and third-party insurers will cover transplants, and when they do, even more people will want them. Whether or not the increase in demand leads to more aggressive procurement strategies, stricter request laws, or the commercialization of human organs, remains to be seen.

CHAPTER 9

THE BIOMORT FACTOR

It *wasn't the philosophers who stimulated cognitive death criteria, it was those who wanted the organs.*
STUART YOUNGNER, M.D.,
Case Western Reserve University

On a shelf behind the desk of Dr. Larry Pitts is a small toy motorcycle. Pasted across the plastic model, in bold letters, is a banner reading DONORCYCLE. Dr. Pitts is the chief of neurology and neurosurgery at San Francisco General Hospital, where Jacesohn Walden spent his last hours. It is from motorcycle accidents that many organ donors come to his hospital.

It is Pitts's responsibility to determine when patients like Jacesohn are dead and organ harvesters can begin their work. He isn't always there to declare death himself, of course, but Pitts has laid down in careful detail the criteria that other physicians in the hospital must follow to set the point in time at which a patient becomes a donor. In fact, Larry Pitts has written the most widely read and popular journal article on brain death. According to Lisa Tulman, transplant coordinator at the University of California, San Francisco, who includes his paper in the curriculum of her transplant liaison training course, Dr. Pitts is "a real friend of transplanting."

That is not an endearment that transplanters reserve for all neurologists, who are of many minds on the subject of brain death and organ donation. In fact, a poll conducted by Brandeis University sociologist Jeffrey Prottas in 1985 revealed that while 90% of all neurosurgeons are comfortable with brain death, more than half of those surveyed felt that medical protocol designed to maintain donatable organs can sometimes conflict with preferred treatment for brain-injured patients.

At the other end of the neurological spectrum from Larry Pitts is Chicago neurosurgeon Richard Nilges, who resents the strong influence of transplant surgery on modern medicine. "The transplant teams are with us," he says, "and the public has come to expect their 'miracles.' Unless there is a technological revolution in the development of artificial organs, the pressure will be increasingly on us, the donors' doctors, to declare our patients 'brain dead,' perhaps even prematurely."

PROFESSIONAL CONFUSION

The coroner's report on Jacesohn Walden states that he was declared "brain dead" at "1130 hours" on March 2, 1987, by a neurologist at San Francisco General Hospital. As it turns out, that was actually the time county coroner Boyd Stephens received a call from the hospital. As required by California law, the caller asked for Stephens's permission to remove Jacesohn's organs for transplanting. Stephens granted permission. That fact is duly noted in his report. Three sentences later is the following entry: "On March 3, at 0031 hours, the deceased was pronounced dead." Walden's chart at San Francisco General says he was declared dead at 11:05 A.M. the previous day.

Well, when was he dead—on Monday or on Tuesday? Was he dead when the neurologist said he was dead or when the coroner said he was dead or when the coroner's report says the hospital says he was dead? Was he "medically" dead at 11:05 on the morning of March 2 (or 11:30), but not "legally" dead until more than twelve hours later at 12:31 A.M., March 3? Was he dead before or after his organs were removed? An official in the coroner's office attempted an explanation. "Brain death requires a second examination at least twelve hours after the first," he said. But if that was the case, why was Walden declared dead after the first examination? Should not the hospital have waited until after the second examination before proceeding with an organ harvest?

Veteran transplant coordinator Amy Peele, who for twelve years has dealt with coroners from Illinois to California, says that many of them, including Stephens, won't declare death until after a respirator has been turned off, which in the Walden case meant after organs had been harvested. That, of course, would imply that Stephens didn't really think Jacesohn Walden was dead when his organs were taken—which, Stephens says, is not the case.

The confusing triple entry in Walden's record is not really that surprising to those who work in or near trauma wards or happen to have followed the "brain death" debates that troubled the medical and legal professions for the twenty years between 1968 and 1988. The often acrimonious struggle between doctors and lawyers to find the point of death has left a wake of distress and confusion that still haunts the medical community. To allay the confusion, the term "biomort" was invented, implying perhaps a third form of being (sort of living, sort of dead). It didn't work. Nor did "neomort," a designation that surfaced in 1974 after a protracted search for something more palatable than "biomort" or "beating-heart cadaver," each considered by primary care physicians to be too offensive for public use. Neither "biomort" nor "neomort" has had wide circulation outside medical/legal circles. "Biomort" first appeared in print in a 1979 legal opinion published in the *Utah Law Review* addressing the "rights of biomorts." The opinion of the author is that biomorts have no rights.

Such opinions notwithstanding, the multiple declaration of Jacesohn Walden's death reflects a whole set of persistent contradictions and confusions that have plagued both professions since brain death became a central medical issue in 1968.

TUCKER V. LOWER

In May of that year a black construction worker named Bruce Tucker fell from a scaffolding in Richmond, Virginia, landing full force on his head. He was rushed to the Medical College of Virginia Hospitals, where he was treated for brain injuries. After opening Tucker's skull to relieve the pressure on his brain, his attending physician noted on his chart that "prognosis for recovery is nil and death imminent."

As it happened, the Medical College of Virginia Hospitals also housed the world-famous heart transplant team headed by Dr. David Hume. On Hume's team was Dr. Richard Lower, who had developed heart transplant techniques with Norman Shumway at the University of Minnesota. Lower, at the time, had a patient named Joseph Klett with severe myocardial infarction. In Lower's opinion, Klett was an ideal candidate for heart transplantation. Lower had been waiting weeks for an ideal donor. Tucker qualified.

Lower, believing that Bruce Tucker was dead by accepted medical standards (i.e., the cessation of all brain functions), removed his healthy beating heart and transplanted it into Joseph Klett. It was the world's seventeenth heart transplant. Christian Barnard had done the first a year earlier.

When Bruce Tucker's brother William read the medical report that said his brother's heart had been removed while it was still beating, he filed a $100,000 damage suit against David Hume and Richard Lower. Tucker claimed that his brother's heart had been removed without the family's permission and before he was dead.

The case, now considered a landmark in both legal *and* medical history, was heard before the Superior Court of Virginia. Before the jury adjourned to deliberate, the judge permitted them to consider all possible causes of death, including "the complete and irreversible loss of all functions of the brain," and to rule that Tucker was dead "whether or not respiration or circulation were spontaneous or were being maintained artificially or mechanically." This was the first time that a judge had given a jury the option of using brain-death criteria as a possible definition of death. Although testimony revealed the fact that William Tucker's business card, showing an address fifteen blocks from the hospital, was found in his brother's wallet and that no telephone call was ever made to obtain permission to harvest organs, in less than an hour the jury brought back a verdict for the defendants.

The *New York Times* headline read, "Virginia Jury Rules That Death Occurs When Brain Dies." The *Washington Post* said, " 'Brain Death' Upheld in Heart Transplant." The American medical community breathed a collective sigh of relief. One of their own had been vindicated and the legal door to organ transplantation had been swung wide open.

After the verdict, Hume and Lower requested that the judge adopt a declaration of death—based on neurological signs—that through case law would become the standard for the whole state of Virginia. The judge refused to do so, saying that "such a radical change" should not be made in court but in the legislature. At the time, however, legislating brain death was not a popular idea among doctors, who generally prefer to keep medical decisions out of the public domain.

Although *Tucker* v. *Lower* made Virginia a safer place to transplant, there remained forty-nine other states where transplant surgeons operated. It seemed inevitable that there would be more attempts to find them guilty of homicide, manslaughter, or wrongful death.

And there were. But as it happened, in most of the cases that followed *Tucker* v. *Lower* the plaintiff was less likely to be a relative of the donor than a criminal defendant accused of killing the donor. The defendant/plaintiff would argue, based on medical records of heartbeat and other vital signs, that the transplant surgeon who removed the heart and other organs had caused the death of the donor ("proximate cause of death" in legalese), *not* the bullet that had entered the deceased's brain and resulted in the cessation of brain functions. While these cases, which appeared from New York to California, were all found in favor of the surgeons, they naturally made the transplant community very nervous.

Shortly after the Tucker trial, thirteen surgeons and physicians met under the auspices of Harvard University and formed the Ad Hoc Committee of the Harvard Medical School to Examine the Definition of Brain Death. While a majority of the Harvard committee were neurologists, two of its most prominent members were surgeons John Merrill and Joseph Murray, who together had performed the first successful kidney transplant at Boston's Peter Brent Brigham hospital in 1954. For Murray and Merrill, an adverse ruling in *Tucker* v. *Lower* would have been devastating. Not only would they have been risking their freedom every time they removed a kidney from a beating-heart cadaver, but in both cases a lifetime of arduous research would have seemed wasted. The Harvard committee agreed that *Tucker* v. *Lower* had been a close call and that it was time to move brain death to a wider, although by no means public, agenda.

Prior to *Tucker* v. *Lower* there *had* been discussions of brain death in the medical community, but only behind closed doors. Records have surfaced of one meeting where brain death was a prominent, though very private, topic. At this meeting, sponsored by (and held at) Ciba House in London, England, in 1965, about two dozen of the world's most prominent transplanters met to discuss the status and future of their specialty. Transcripts of the meeting indicate that surgeons were not of one mind on the subject of brain death. Sir Roy Calne, for example, stated, in response to brain-death criteria proposed by Dr. Guy Alexandre of Brussels, that "although Dr. Alexandre's criteria are medically persuasive, according to traditional definitions of death, he is, in fact, removing kidneys from live donors. I feel that if a person has a heartbeat, he cannot be regarded as a cadaver." Strangely enough, Calne seemed more concerned about transplant surgeons' reputation within the medical community than within society at large. "Any modification of the means of diagnosing death to facilitate transplantation," he said, "will cause the whole procedure to fall into disrepute with the rest of the profession."

Dr. Thomas Starzl, then at the University of Colorado, was also hestitant to declare a person dead if his or her heart was beating. "Initially, the fear that the quality of terminal care provided for the donor might be lessened caused us to speak out against the pronouncement of death in the presence of a heartbeat," he recalls. But by 1969 Starzl would radically change his position. "Later experience convinced us that such anxieties were unfounded." Starzl has since become one of the most aggressive transplanters in the field and an outspoken supporter of brain-death statutes.

By mid-1968 all fifty state legislatures had received drafts of the Uniform Anatomical Gift Act. It was therefore an auspicious time to take the next step and introduce a brain-death statute. The best way to do that, the Harvard committee felt, was to propose a suitable protocol for distinguishing patients with "total irreversible loss of all brain function" from those who were merely comatose. In August of 1968 the committee released a list of criteria for declaring death. They proposed the following tests and recommended that anyone failing all four should be declared dead:

1. Unreceptivity and unresponsiveness
2. No movement or breathing
3. No reflexes
4. Flat electroencephalogram (EEG)

To each general criterion was attached a short explanation of the tests that should be applied to determine the condition. The Harvard committee also recommended that before final pronouncement of death, all tests be repeated twenty-four hours after brain death is diagnosed, and that an EEG be used only as a confirmatory technology, "when available." Any patients suffering from hypothermia (extremely low body temperature) or carrying traces of barbiturates in their blood should not be declared dead according to the committee, who were familiar with several cases where supercooled or barbiturated patients, displaying all the symptoms of brain death, had eventually recovered to live normal lives.

The Harvard criteria, as they came to be known, were published in the *Journal of the American Medical Association* under the title "A Definition of Irreversible Coma"—a surprising choice of headline for anyone who had come to accept "coma" as a *living* state that could in no way be equated, legally or medically, with death. Despite that fact, the Harvard committee's opening sentence read, "Our primary purpose is to define irreversible *coma* as a *new* criterion for death." (Emphasis added.)

The committee gave two reasons why the definition of death had to be changed. The first was to relieve the burden placed on "patients who suffer permanent loss of intellect, on their families, on the hospitals and on those in need of hospital beds occupied by comatose patients." The second reason was that "obsolete criteria for the definition of death can lead to controversy in obtaining organs for transplantation." In light of the Tucker trial and how it could have turned out, that, of course, was an understatement. It was unquestionably the first motive that rallied so many physicians to support the Harvard criteria. But it was the second that gave them pause.

"If we accept the argument," said Richard Nilges, "that the benefits of organ transplantation far outweigh the potential harm to donor patients, we accept the possible killing of innocent people for the good of recipient patients. Where will we stop; where the healthy and strong may do what they like with the weak and the sick?"

Others felt that transplanters were too conspicuously involved in brain-death deliberations. Earl Walker, an Albuquerque, New Mexico, neurosurgeon and medical historian who has written a book on brain death, remembers the early days. "At first, transplant surgeons were very visible. But people became skeptical about their biases, so their input into brain-death criteria was minimized. However, to people who worked closely with the issue, the role of transplant surgeons was always evident.''

The truth was that transplanters were very eager to have the protection that brain-death legislation would afford them, but didn't need to stay on the front line of the issue. In fact, they knew it was unwise to do so. Neurosurgeons and neurologists needed brain-death statutes far more than transplanters did and their cause was more noble. Transplanters, therefore, could sit back and rely on a much more compelling rationale than organ availability. And that's exactly what they did. While the debate on brain death swirled around their specialty, they focused their energy on aggressive public and professional education programs aimed at enhancing organ procurement.

Transplant surgeons would occasionally surface in the brain-death debate to argue a point of medicine, but rarely in a public arena. At a fairly obscure brain-death case in New York State (*New York* v. *Sulsona*), for example, a group of surgeons testified that kidneys from donors whose deaths were caused by cardiac arrest or respiratory failure had an 88% failure rate, while kidneys from brain-dead donors were, they said, equal in quality to kidneys from the living (with only a 10% failure rate). The testimony paid off for transplanters. New York State, due to effective anti-brain-death lobbying efforts, had been unable to pass a brain-death statute, so surgeons and lawyers had to rely on case law for their protection. *New York* v. *Sulsona* now offers some of that protection.

INVOKING THE POPE

At the end of medical articles one normally finds a long list of references, at times even a bibliography. In 1968 there was certainly a sizable volume of medical literature on death and dying that could have been cited after any report on the subject. At the bottom of the Harvard committee's article was one citation:

1. Pius XII, "The Prolongation of Life," *Pope Speaks* 4 (1958): 393–398.

During the previous year Pope Pius XII had made a speech in which he had pronounced that doctors were not obligated to make extraordinary resuscitative efforts with very sick patients. "Normally one is held to use only ordinary means," said the Pope, "that is to say, means that do not involve any grave burden for oneself or another." Perhaps members of the committee were anticipating some resistance to their ideas from Catholics. They certainly got it from Paul Byrne, a pediatric neurologist, Roman Catholic, and lifelong crusader for the repeal of brain-death statutes, who believes the Pope's declaration was misinterpreted and abused by the Harvard committee.

In 1975 Byrne treated a young boy named Joseph Van Dyke, who was admitted to his hospital with serious head injuries. Van Dyke was placed on a ventilator, where he remained in a comatose state. Six weeks later an EEG was taken and interpreted as being "consistent with cerebral death." Byrne, however, refused to declare him dead. Joseph Van Dyke recovered from his coma and is today a healthy, normal teenager.

"That's when I started studying brain death," recalls Byrne, who today travels to state capitals with Joseph Van Dyke to testify at hearings on brain-death legislation. Together they claim to have stopped bills in at least two states. Byrne says that the very concept of brain death reflects "a basic shift in the practice of medicine . . . and any legislation which furthers, aids, or gives color of legitimacy to this change opens the door to dehumanization . . . by allowing the lives of the innocent to be hazarded without necessity." To Byrne, brain death, as defined by its proponents, "implies a strict materialism . . . reducing the life of a human person to a putative organic function of material brain.'' He is absolutely convinced that brain-death legislation is a conspiracy of transplanters—a theory that has done little to enhance his cause or credibility.

Byrne says that society does not understand ''the issue sufficiently to have given informed consent.'' He has since spent much of his time mobilizing and instructing opponents, particularly right-to-life and pro-life organizations, on the fine points of neurology. ''We have been told,'' he tells them, ''that it is now possible to sustain for months or years a 'mechanically profuse cadaver.' It is contended that this body with its regular pulse, its near normal warmth and coloration, its continuous output of sweat and urine, is not a body at all but a carefully and expensively maintained corpse.''

Pro-life advocates, with some prodding from Paul Byrne, have come to see brain-death statutes not only as a convenience for transplanters but also as a ''foot-in-the-door'' for euthanasia. There is also some fear in pro-life and conservative Catholic circles that brain-death laws will one day be used to add legal support to first-trimester abortion. The argument they anticipate is that since zygotes have no brains, they are de facto brain dead.

Byrne and the right-to-life lobby argue that simple loss of brain function is not sufficient to declare death because there is no way to be absolutely certain, with *any* criteria, that loss of brain function is permanent or ''irreversible.'' According to Byrne and his supporters, before death should be declared—for reasons other than the old and accepted cardiopulmonary cessation—the brain must be organically destroyed as it might be ''if someone's head had been completely crushed by a truck, or vaporized by a nuclear blast, or his brain had been dissolved by a massive injection of sulfuric acid.''

''Well, I haven't had many cases like that recently,'' says Ron Cranford, a Minneapolis neurologist who actively supports the passage of brain-death statutes. Cranford dismisses Byrne and his followers as ''pro-life zealots.''

STATUTES

The first brain-death statute was passed in the state of Kansas in 1970, about a year after the Tucker trial ended. The bill passed with surprisingly little public attention or opposition, although news of its passage did bring the issue to the forefront of medical and legal discussions. Within both professions, now joined by religious and bioethical leaders, there remained nagging confusions and uncertainties about the "brain centered" concept of life and death. Harvard committee chairman Henry Beecher remarked just before the Kansas bill passed, "Almost every doctor on the East Coast has accepted irreversible brain damage as the criterion for death, whereas most West Coast physicians do not, for fear of suits." In fact, the issue was not quite so neatly divided at the Mississippi; for closer to home, in fact right at his own university, Beecher was hearing from Professor David Rutstein, who openly expressed concern over "this major ethical change that has occurred right before our eyes . . . with so little public discussion of its significance."

The Kansas statute, at least for a while after it passed, caused "more problems than it solved," according to Alexander Capron, at one time a University of Pennsylvania law professor and now a lawyer at the University of Southern California. It stipulated that death should be pronounced before a respirator was removed and, of course "before any vital organ is removed for transplantation." The bill as worded gave the impression that there were two separate kinds of death. And that confusion was compounded by the fact that the bill read as if it had been drafted for the purpose of assisting organ transplantation. When the state of Maryland passed the same law, the public outcry was so great that the legislature amended the statute to remove alternative provisions for declaring death.

For the next five years, one after another, states passed brain-death laws, each a little different than the ones before it. Virginia's, passed in 1973, required the declaration of two physicians, one a neurologist or neurosurgeon, and added a new test to the criteria—the so-called "apnea test," wherein the respirator is removed for a short period of time to be certain that there is no spontaneous breathing. This test did not make transplanters a bit happy, because while the test is in progress no oxygen is reaching the organs they hope to remove.

The New Mexico and Alaska statutes, passed in 1973 and 1974, respectively, are similar to the Kansas law. And Oregon's 1975 law actually simplified the definition by saying that "when a physician acts to determine that a person is dead, he may make such a determination if irreversible cessation of spontaneous respiration and circulatory function *or* irreversible cessation of spontaneous brain function exists."

The one problem common to all six of the statutes that had been legislated by 1975 was that each contained two separate definitions of death and implied that it was up to the attending physician to chose which he or she wanted to employ. And since one of the definitions left the heart beating, public suspicion persisted that death was being redefined for the benefit of organ transplanters.

In 1981 the U.S. Congress became interested in the brain-death controversy and requested the President's Commission for the Study of Ethical Problems in Medicine to draft yet another uniform brain-death statute. For eighteen months a committee of the commission, chaired by Alex Capron, considered every conceivable definition of death, ranging from the eighteenth-century notion that putrification was the only sure sign, to more contemporary and radical proposals that death also be defined as the permanent loss of cognitive ("higher") brain functions (now known as "cortical," or "cognitive," death).

From the start, however, the commissioners were determined to be conservative and to produce a model statute that would be suitable for physicians, understood by the laity, and acceptable to theologians from the major religious groups in America. What they eventually endorsed was the Uniform Definition of Death Act (UDDA), a revision of the Uniform Brain Death Act (UBDA), which had been drafted at a special commission meeting in Chicago held with key delegates of the American Medical Association (AMA), the American Bar Association (ABA), and the National Conference on Uniform State Laws.

With a cautiously worded definition, including "irreversible cessation of all functions of the brain, *including the brain stem*," the drafters hoped to expand support for the bill. The brain stem, also known as the "ascending reticular formation," is a Y-shaped cluster of nerve cells and fibers located directly under the cerebellum. As well as acting as a sort of command center for both cerebral hemispheres, the brain stem also controls the sleep-awake function and stimulates such vital involuntary activities as breathing. It is to brain stem activity that neurologists and neurosurgeons look for the last symptoms of human life.

"When I saw 'including the brain stem,' I thought it was ridiculous," recalls Ron Cranford. "We were in effect saying the same thing *three* times. Their rejoinder was that it was the best way to distinguish brain death from the 'permanent vegetative state.' I said I thought that was stupid." Although "including the brain stem" seemed redundant to others as well, the commission felt that to avoid the misconception that brain death meant only loss of *cognitive* function, they should add the redundancy. "Fortunately, they didn't heed my advice," recalls Cranford, "and it worked. The wording made it very clear that we didn't mean Karen Quinlan could be declared dead and harvested."

By 1981 brain-death laws had been passed or ruled into law by twenty-six state legislatures, ten state supreme courts, and thirteen other nations. Versions of the law varied from one-sentence statements to longer statutes that included detailed stipulations and religious exclusions. The UDDA had, however, become the most widely accepted legal standard for determining death.

THE BERGER CASE

Within months of the President's Commission report, an incident in New York State placed the whole brain-death debate once again in high relief and gave the prolegislation forces a classic case-study to prove their point that America needed brain-death laws.

On March 23, 1982, Richard Berger, a nineteen-year-old boy, was admitted to the Smithtown (Long Island) General Hospital with a bullet wound in the head. He had no reflex responses and was unable to breathe without a respirator. His pupils were dilated and fixed. There was no response to light or painful stimuli and his EEG was flat.

"Is he dead?" his father asked.

"He is brain dead," the doctor answered.

"Is he *legally* dead?" asked the father.

"I don't know," replied the doctor. "I am not a lawyer."

The next six days were pure hell for Richard Berger's parents, who watched doctors, lawyers, district attorneys, and transplant surgeons squabble over the status and future of their son, who lay comatose and respirated in an intensive care ward. Physicians were convinced he was dead, but refused to declare it until his parents either obtained a court order to do so or agreed to donate his organs for transplantation. Because there was no brain-death statute in New York, the only protection the doctors felt they had was the Uniform Anatomical Gift Act, which allows the removal of organs from the brain dead. The district attorney warned Richard's parents that the defendant in Richard's murder trial would surely argue that *they* had killed him, not the assailant's bullet.

On the sixth day Richard had a heart attack, dashing his parents' secret hopes for a miraculous recovery. At that point they were again confronted with the question of organ donation, but this time they were told that if they didn't decide soon, the organs would go to waste. They agreed to donate.

In New York State powerful Catholic and orthodox Jewish lobbies have effectively kept brain-death statutes off the books.

The result has been a real reluctance on the part of doctors or family members to "pull the plug," even on patients who would clearly be declared brain dead a few miles away in a neighboring state. "As things stand now, withdrawal of life support is homicide" in New York State, Robert Adams, district attorney of Rensselaer County, told a statewide conference on the Legal and Ethical Aspects of Treatment of the Critically and Terminally Ill. Adams further alarmed the physicians in attendance by adding that "there are D.A.s in the state anxious to pursue such charges." Because brain death remains so controversial in New York, and undefined by statute, there is much less transplant surgery done there than the population would warrant. Most New Yorkers who require transplants travel to Boston or Pittsburgh for their surgery.

RADICALS AND HERETICS

Paul Byrne has had his theses published, once in the *Journal of the American Medical Association* (almost eleven years after publication of the Harvard criteria) and again in the relatively obscure *Gonzaga Law Review* (Spokane, Washington). Few of his contemporaries in medicine, however, ever took him or his position very seriously. Some of that response is probably deserved. Byrne's position is after all, extreme and heretical, medically if not theologically.

However, in 1983 Byrne offered an intriguing caveat to the laity. He said that the medical community, having sought and gained "a determination of death which enables a physician to treat a body as a corpse at the earliest moment possible," would begin to push the envelope further back, by defining as dead people who have lost only cognitive functions or are in a diagnosed "permanent vegetative state." "Within a year of any universal acceptance of a general criterion of death based on irreversible function of the brain," Byrne predicted, "the drive for 'cortical death' will be fully under way."

Right now there are about 10,000 people hospitalized in the

U.S. who have been diagnosed as permanently vegetative, a condition that brain-injured patients often regress to when they haven't recovered from a regular coma in about thirty days. As alarmist as Byrne's prediction seems, there are some disturbing intellectual fragments scattered through the literature suggesting that people in a permanent vegetative state should join the ranks of the biomorts.

Henry Beecher, chairman of the Harvard committee and still considered the godfather of brain-death criteria, does not go quite that far. But two years after drafting the Harvard definition, he did list the qualities he considered essential to humanity, without which human life no longer existed: "The individual personality, his conscious life, his uniqueness, his capacity for remembering, judging, reasoning, acting, enjoying, worrying and so on." Beecher believed these functions took place entirely in the brain, and therefore "when the brain no longer functions . . . so also is the individual destroyed; he no longer exists as a person. He is dead." All the functions Beecher listed, however, take place in the cerebral cortex, none in the brain stem.

In their landmark article, published in the late 1972 by the *University of Pennsylvania Law Review*, Alexander Capron and Leon Kass looked to the future of organ transplantation: "If more organs are needed than can be legally obtained, the question of whether the benefits conferred by transplantation justify the risks associated with [a] broader definition of death should be addressed directly, rather than by trying to subsume it under the question 'what is death?'

"Such a direct confrontation with the issue," they concluded, "could lead to a discussion about the standards and procedures under which organs might be taken from persons *near* death, or even those still quite alive, at their own option or that of relatives, physicians or representatives of the state." (Emphasis added.)

As we have seen, radical nostrums get tossed about professional communities long before they ever reach the public. Of course, the purpose in keeping such deeply controversial proposals under wraps for as long as possible is to allow time for consensus to form in the profession and to be certain that when new ideas and definitions do reach the public, they are respectfully packaged and endorsed by organizations like the AMA, ABA, and as many other professional and religious groups as possible. Above all, the proponents must be braced for the reaction that will inevitably follow.

By 1987 the concept of cortical death had been broached, although not yet proposed, by Beecher, Capron, Kass, and others. Capron moved the concept one step closer to a proposal in a recently published treatise written primarily for doctors and lawyers called *Medico-Legal Aspects of Critical Care*. "There are two possible solutions to the problem of shortage of useful human organs," says Capron: "(1) promulgating a statute, with special procedures to prevent abuse, that would permit organs to be removed from '*pre*-mortem organ donors' and (2) allowing people to request that if they are dying their organs be 'harvested' at a point in the dying process *before* it would be appropriate to bury or mourn them, *even though they are not dead by definition*." (Emphasis added.)

Capron is influential. As his cautious suggestions gain respectability, others are willing to shift the locus of death closer to the living state. Stuart Youngner, a psychiatrist at Case Western Reserve University in Cleveland, Ohio, for example, has studied and written about the psychosocial implications of organ transplantation, and now says that since "we are willing to declare patients dead when there is a considerable amount of life left in their bodies," we should broaden our definition of death to include *cognitive* death. "Once consciousness is irreversibly lost," he says, reminiscent of Beecher, "the person is lost. What remains is a mindless organism. The innate integration of vegetative functions cannot be used as a necessary and sufficient condition for life." What happens after the loss of personhood, Youngner says, is "the demise of a body that has outlived its owner." A person in such a state, according to Youngner, should be declared dead. Youngner's articles, like Capron's, are widely read in the transplant community.

Capron, Veatch, Youngner, and proponents of cortical death deny that they are changing, or ever intended to change, the "definition of death." Death is death, they say. It is the point in the dying process (the locus) at which life ends and death begins that they are trying to pinpoint.

The Task Force on Death and Dying put it this way: "To ask 'What is death?' is to ask similarly 'What makes living things alive?' To understand death as the transition between something alive and that same something dead presupposes that one understands the difference between 'alive' and 'dead'—that one understands what it is that dies."

CHAPTER 10

BACKSTAGE/ FRONTSTAGE

The problems came when transplantation shifted from magic to commerce.

THOMAS STARZL, M.D.,
University of Pittsburgh

In early September of 1987, the University of Pittsburgh hosted the first annual International Transplant Forum. Of course, international meetings of transplant physicians, surgeons, and coordinators had been held before in different parts of the world. And there already existed at least one international organization of transplanters, the Transplant Society. But this meeting was unique in that the week-long agenda included a full two days of nonmedical (ethical, religious, political, and economic) discussions. The forum was also held in tandem with a convention of 300 transplant recipients from around the world who had recently formed a consumer-oriented group called the Transplant Recipients International Organization. The combined event was promoted as a tribute to Thomas Starzl, Pitt's chief of transplant surgery.

Here gathered with their former patients, for the first time anywhere, were the major players in the organ transplant complex—Keith Reemtsma, chief of surgery at Columbia University; Francis D. Moore, Harvard's patriarch of transplantation; Gene Pierce, founder and director of the United Network for Organ Sharing (UNOS); Felix Rapaport, editor of *Transplantation Proceedings*; Jean-François Borel from the Sandoz Chemical

175

Company in Switzerland; Paul Terasaki from UCLA; Carl Groth from the Karolinska Institute in Stockholm; Oscar Salvatierra, Jr., director of the largest kidney transplant unit in the world, at the University of California; and the University of Minnesota's John Najarian, who came "not to honor Starzl, but to read a paper." The Starzl-Najarian rivalry was by then legendary, so no one was surprised when Najarian left the forum shortly after reading his paper. Although many *had* come to honor Starzl, most were there to hear other scientists read papers or to consult with immunologists and histologists, hear religious leaders reveal their positions on organ donation, and, perhaps most poignant of all, to meet again some of the people that had benefited from their technology.

Pittsburgh, Pennsylvania, home for the largest transplant unit in the world, was an appropriate location for the first International Transplant Forum. Credit for Pittsburgh's stature as a transplant mecca must also go to Henry Bahnson, the university's modest but aggressive chief of surgery, who in 1981 convinced Tom Starzl not to move from the University of Colorado to UCLA, but to come to Pittsburgh instead. Though at the time some physicians and hospital administrators in Los Angeles were relieved not to have such a controversial surgeon in their midst they undoubtedly now wish that Starzl had moved south instead of east. His astounding success with patients no one else would transplant has attracted more talent and more patients to Pittsburgh than Bahnson or the university ever bargained for. Starzl didn't do it alone, of course, but if he hadn't been there, it is doubtful Pittsburgh would have become a world capital of transplantation, matched in American stature only by the University of Minnesota —a not always friendly rival on the playing fields of transplant philosophy and practice.

BREAKTHROUGHS AND WAR STORIES

During the week in Pittsburgh, some major new breakthroughs in transplant science were announced, among them a new solution that would preserve livers for twenty-four hours; a powerful and sensitive scanning machine that could detect the earliest signs of organ rejection; an immunosuppressive drug a thousand times stronger than cyclosporine; and a high-speed multiple-organ retrieval that allowed transplanters to take vital hearts, livers, and kidneys from donors who had previously been impossible to harvest. But breakthroughs are revealed at most scientific and medical conventions; in fact, many are announced in the mass media before the conventions even take place. It is the war stories and open expressions of attitude that make a gathering of titans worth attending.

At a panel on government policy, for example, Dr. Ross Anthony, an official of the Health Care Financing Administration, offered this anecdote on the hard choices faced by healthcare policymakers in Washington: "When I was working several years ago in a small rural clinic in Nepal, a man appeared one day carrying his four-year-old son on his back. They had come from a village five days away and the boy was very sick. The only way to save him would be to radio for a plane to fly in to a dirt strip and take him out to a hospital in Katmandu. And even at that I didn't think he had a very good chance of living.

"Now, I had an annual budget for the whole clinic of about twenty thousand dollars and it would have cost me over five hundred dollars to fly the boy out. For five hundred dollars I could inoculate every child in four nearby valleys against diseases that would surely kill hundreds of them. Now, what was I to do?" Without hesitation Tom Starzl, who was moderating the panel, grabbed the microphone and said, "Fly him out."

Therein lies one of the most basic moral conflicts in contemporary American healthcare. On one side stands the policymaker who must decide where and when to appropriate scarce resources, balancing heroic but expensive technologies that may rescue a few against the mundane preventive measures that protect the many. On the other stands the noble surgeon whose Hippocratic vows oblige him to save the dying patient when he appears and to heal others when they get sick.

UNDERCURRENTS

Veteran transplanters like Felix Rapaport, Keith Reemtsma, Fred Belzer, and Francis D. "Franny" Moore, the Harvard Medical School surgeon emeritus who has written a book on transplant medicine, bring to any forum a rich and clear sense of history, and in their open dialogues reveal the world behind the scenes of organ transplantation, a world less heroic perhaps than the image created by hospital PR teams, but one with its own curious excitement and drama.

There were some subtle, unscheduled themes that surfaced at the forum. A topic that almost seemed to dominate the agenda, at times, was xenografting—the transplanting of organs from one species to another, from subhuman primates to man, for instance. Although there were no major papers scheduled on xenografting, the subject arose in workshops, speeches, and discussions. It seemed as if a once-abandoned dream was being revived—spontaneously. Reemtsma and Starzl, who had been derided by medical peers and religious leaders less than twenty-five years earlier for placing the kidneys and livers of chimpanzees and baboons into the bodies of living men and women, were now able to joke about what they were almost disrobed for doing.

It was at a plenary session of the forum that Reemtsma confessed before a thousand people that in 1964, while practicing at Tulane University, he had hidden a human patient in a room over the laundry, where snoopy reporters wouldn't find him. Why? Because the patient had been transplanted with the kidneys of a chimpanzee. "I invited David Hume and Tom Starzl in to visit one day," Reemtsma told his peers. "They seemed shocked at what I had done. 'What the *hell* are you doing?' said Hume. But both of them went home, Hume to Virginia and Starzl to Colorado, and began looking for primates. Hume looked everywhere for chimps. Starzl looked in the yellow pages and stopped at 'B' for baboons." The story brought the house down. A forbidden experiment, which might then have ended the medical careers of three great surgeons, now seemed acceptable.

Twenty-five years of acute organ shortage had done a lot to make xenografting a respectable possibility. The agenda is no longer hidden. In 1987 Reemtsma applied to the Institute Review Board at Columbia University to begin an experimental series transplanting chimpanzee hearts either as boosters (hearts implanted beside the ailing human heart) or as bridges (hearts temporarily transplanted) in humans waiting for a human heart.

A CONCOCTION OF MEDICINE AND POLITICS

Billed as a major speaker at the forum was Sen. Albert Gore, Jr. Although Gore is a political friend, even hero, to some in the transplant community, few were surprised or even disappointed when he sent his aide, Jerold Mande, in his stead. Gore had recently announced his candidacy for President, and Mande was known by most in attendance as the brains and impetus behind the Organ Transplant Act of 1984.

It was inevitable that at least some federal legislators would take an interest in organ transplantation. It is rife with the kind of dramatic emotional imagery that is bound to attract public attention. Interest in transplantation seems to have arisen almost simultaneously on both sides of the hill, but no single legislator has played a larger role in the issues surrounding it than Gore, a studious junior senator from Tennessee who has, since entering public life, enjoyed the challenge of esoteric technologies and complex policy issues. Transplantation was, according to Jerold Mande, "a natural area of concern" for his boss.

Gore first became aware of the controversies and potentials of organ transplanting at a 1982 Ohio State University conference on end-stage renal disease. There he came to the conclusion that kidney transplants were a cost-effective way to get people off the terribly expensive federal dialysis program in a manner that also made most patients stronger and more productive, sometimes able to return to work.

But like so many other public figures who have taken a personal interest in transplantation, Gore was finally drawn to action by the drama of an individual case—and what could be more dramatic than a kid who needs a liver? And what a perfect kid was Jamie Fiske. Like all of us, Gore watched with amazement while the dramatic and successful transplant involving a beautiful young child was played out before the nation in bold relief. Within hours after the operation, Gore and Mande began drafting legislation.

Then, in January of 1983, the senator received a letter from the parents of a little boy in Tennessee named Brandon Hall. Brandon was going to die any day, the letter said, unless he got a liver. Gore invited the Halls to attend hearings on the bill he and Mande had drafted and were about to introduce. Brandon came too and the hearing room was packed with media, including crews from all four networks. The Halls's impassioned testimony aired, and later that same evening Brandon got his liver. But Brandon didn't do as well as Jamie Fiske, alas. He rejected the liver. A few days later he was given a second transplant, but he also rejected that and eventually died.

From the standpoint of political mileage, however, it doesn't really matter whether a media darling makes it or not. In fact, in some cases it's better if he or she doesn't. In 1987, for example, Ronnie De Sillers gave the media and at least one politician several days of continuous dramatic coverage, beginning the morning that $5,000 was stolen from a fund set up by his schoolmates in Florida to pay for a trip to Pittsburgh. Within hours after the story hit the wires, there was $450,000 in Ronnie's bank account, including a check for $1,000 signed by Ronald Reagan, a photo of which ran on the front page of most every newspaper in the country. It took four livers before young Ronnie succumbed. It was a drama that kept him, his mother, his surgeons, the University of Pittsburgh, and the president of the United States on the front page for over a week. Few outside the medical community ever questioned whether retransplanting the same patient four times was sound medical practice or whether this kind of publicity was, in the long run, healthy for transplantation. It was certainly healthy for political and surgical careers.

When legislators became interested in transplantation, transplanters became interested in Washington, although begrudgingly so. As much as they disliked any government interference in medical practice, surgeons and hospital administrators saw congressional curiosity about transplantation as an opportunity to improve organ procurement systems, increase research funding, and extend the entitlement of transplantation from kidneys to other ("extrarenal") organs.

Throughout the early 1980s several omnibus transplantation bills were submitted to Congress. Only one, however, made it through hearings and onto the floor of both houses. HR 4080 was sponsored by Gore, who said, ironically enough, that the bill was designed to match donors and recipients based on medical need, "not on who has the cutest face or the most money." Actually, HR 4080 was a composite of previous legislative attempts on the part of Edward Kennedy, Orrin Hatch, and Mark Andrews in the Senate and Henry Waxman in the House to provide some federal assistance for, and regulation of, organ transplanting: After the Brandon Hall show, future hearings on the Gore bill were well attended by transplant surgeons, transplant coordinators, organ procurement officials, AMA lawyers, hospital administrators, parents with dying children, and others with special interests.

Transplants had by then become a reliable media sop. The best formula was still a very sick child, a tearful parent or two, and a powerful public figure. Even Sen. Jesse Helms, arguably the most conservative member of either house, whom one might expect to eschew any suggestion of federal support for healthcare, stepped briefly into the transplant spotlight. At a hearing before the Senate Committee on Labor and Human Resources held on October 20, 1983, Helms barged into the committee room with three constituents, Mr. and Mrs. Rick Brooks and their baby boy, Joshua, from Laurinburg, North Carolina. Helms asked to be placed at the top of the agenda. His message was urgent.

Little Joshua Brooks was suffering from biliary atresia, a

terminal condition that can be cured only with a liver transplant. Helms introduced the family to the committee, gave a quick and redundant primer on organ transplantation, said that the nation had to do something about little Joshua, and ran back to the Agriculture Committee, which was also in session. Chairman Orrin Hatch then held little Joshua on his lap, while cameras flashed and whirred and Mr. and Mrs. Brooks made an impassioned plea for their child's life. When Sen. Mark Andrews accused Hatch of playing to the cameras, the hearing room was filled with laughter. And the cameras kept rolling. Dying children had become political theater.

CENTER STAGE

The Reagan years were boom years for transplantation. New centers opened in almost every state, the number of operations grew exponentially year by year, and transplantation became an increasingly hot topic—particularly in the media. And there has never in history been a more media-conscious or media-savvy administration than Ronald Reagan's. The White House press office quickly saw that becoming identified with an individual transplant crisis was, in the early 1980s, a perfect way for anyone's imagemaker to grab a little easy ink for the boss. Drama, pathos, and heroism were built in; all one needed was a good case and a good face—baby, parent, or politician. It didn't much matter.

Early in the first Reagan administration, Michael Batten, a pugnacious public relations specialist in the White House public liaison office, was assigned to be point man on organ transplanting. When word reached the transplant community (consumers included) that there was a sympathetic ear at the 1600 Pennsylvania Avenue, Batten's phone rang off the hook. He called his office "the body shop" and for six years used his access to the Reagans to perform some miracles for a few desperate Americans and, in the process, to bolster the President's image as a charitable humanitarian leader. Before he left the White House in March of 1987, Batten says, he fielded more than 1,500 requests for Presidential intervention. Most often the calls were from parents hoping that Reagan or the First Lady would make a public appeal for a new organ for their little child, or cudgel an insurance carrier (public or private) into covering a particular transplant. Batten, acting on behalf of the President, leaned relentlessly on surgeons, hospital administrators, insurance executives, Air Force colonels, and other decision makers.

Batten relished his power. "All I had to do," he says, "was call a state official or insurance executive and say, 'I guess I'm going to have to tell Mrs. Reagan,' and it was enough to get an operation covered or have an Air Force jet rolled out in the middle of the night to speed a dying kid to a transplant center." If the Air Force balked, as they once did, Batten simply shifted tactics and said, "Do this one for the Gipper," and the plane was airborne. The next morning headlines across the nation would read: PRESIDENT SAVES CHILD WITH LIVER DISEASE. It was great press and it was basically free.

Things didn't always work out quite so well for the beneficiary as they did for the White House. For example, when Thomas Starzl made a personal appeal to the White House on behalf of a forty-four-year-old suburbanite from Detroit named Judy Tazelaar, Batten rose to the occasion, assuring Starzl that the federal government would pay for her surgery. The next day Tazelaar, who had been waiting for months for a new liver, was transplanted. (WHITE HOUSE HELPS PAVE WAY FOR OPERATION, read a Pittsburgh headline.) The problem was that Tazelaar wasn't really eligible for either Medicare or Medicaid, and state and federal bureaucrats were unwilling to make an exception, even for the President. Starzl's hospital got stuck for $100,000. Batten's response: "We'll just have to ask the folks in Pittsburgh to do one for the Gipper." And before that wisecrack landed him in trouble, he said, "I don't really want the hospital to get caught on this one . . . but the point is she's alive." And, of course, the boss had some more good publicity.

Batten could also play hardball. When Medicaid officials in Massachusetts refused to come up with $180,000 to pay for Sara Brookwood's liver transplant, Batten called Gov. Edward J. King and told him that if the state didn't pay for the transplant, there would be a full-page ad in the *Boston Globe*, signed by Brookwood's father, saying "the Governor of Massachusetts is responsible for my daughter's death." That afternoon King's office directed Medicaid to cover the operation.

Batten's action and King's compliance created a precedent that has been followed several times since, where the family of a transplant patient recruits the President or another powerful politician to intervene on their behalf. "We come in and make them look like dogs," boasted Batten in 1984. "They always knuckle under." With similar bravado, Batten was able to persuade the entire Texas legislature to pass a special bill appropriating $41,000 to cover a transplant for Ashley Bailey, who had become an overnight media darling when the President mentioned her on his Saturday afternoon radio broadcast.

A NEAR VETO

Despite an expressed compassion for transplant patients, "the administration never liked the idea of legislation benefiting organ transplanting," remembers Jerold Mande. Indeed Dr. Edward Brandt, assistant secretary for health of the Department of Health and Human Services, and Carol K. Davis of the same agency's Health Care Financing Administration were both dispatched to the hill on February 9, 1984, to express strong opposition to the Gore bill. Although Nancy and Ronald Reagan seemed willing to do anything for a child in need of a new organ, says Mande, "Reagan did everything he could to discourage or block the Gore bill. He even tried to obviate any federal legislation by forming the American Council on Transplantation [ACT]."

ACT, as conceived by the administration, was to be a private nonprofit federation of transplant surgeons, organ procurement agencies, transplant coordinators, tissue typers, and others in the medical community whose aim it would be to improve the organ procurement system. Shortly after it was formed, Surgeon General C. Everett Koop awarded ACT a $100,000 seed grant, which gave him an opportunity to say that he, too, thought the whole business of organ and tissue procurement belonged in the private sector. At first Koop found it difficult to attract many of the organizations or leaders in the transplant community into the federation. In fact, many of the 300 organizations Reagan hoped would participate actually boycotted the first meeting, some stating that ACT was simply a front for the administration set up to block Albert Gore's legislation.

According to Mande, "ACT *was* a front, designed to create private-sector legitimacy and frustrate *all* legislative efforts, not just Gore's. But when ACT board members realized what was happening, Oscar Salvatierra [then president of the American Society of Transplant Surgeons] and three other prominent directors resigned on December 26, 1983, leaving Gary Friedlaender, at the time an obscure osteopathic surgeon from Yale, alone to face the public embarrassment of leading the administration's stalking horse."

By the time it came before Congress, the Gore bill was watered down somewhat to maximize its political appeal in both houses, where it passed overwelmingly. Despite his vocal opposition and active efforts to subvert the legislation, the President signed the Organ Transplant Act into law in October of 1984. A veto would certainly have been overridden.

In 1986 the White House was again faced with an opportunity to do something really substantial for organ transplantation. But again, Reagan balked. The Department of Health and Human Services granted $750,000 to the United Network for Organ Sharing (UNOS), which had been selected to implement the national computerized organ-sharing program recommended by the administration-appointed National Task Force on Organ Transplantation. In 1987 Reagan removed the UNOS appropriation from the 1988 fiscal-year budget. UNOS was a private nonprofit organization, the President argued, that could survive on membership dues and the $200 fee charged for every patient listed on the national waiting list.

The administration had long before chosen to ignore its own Task Force, which, upon completion of research in April of 1986, recommended various degrees of federal support for transplants. Not only was the White House "unable" to find a room for the Task Force to hold a press conference and announce its findings, but when the Task Force staff eventually found a room on Capitol Hill, the administration stayed away. Charles T. Kline, spokesman for the Department of Health and Human Services, told *The New York Times* that since most of the Task Force's recommendations were addressed to private industry, doctors, and hospitals, no response was required from the White House.

Senator Gore fired an angry salvo down Pennsylvania Avenue, describing the President as "breathtakingly hypocritical" on the issue of transplantation. "For the White House to seize on transplant cases that already have received publicity as a way of generating good press for itself is one thing," said Gore on February 18, 1987. "To then turn around, and in the dead of night, strip the budget of the money needed to keep the entire donor system running, inspires utter contempt."

Batten, who called Gore and his legislation "silly and mischievous" and who referred to the organ procurement organizations that supported it as "giblet gravy groups," defended his boss's case-by-case approach to the problem of organ scarcity. "We aren't going to sit around and wait for policy," he said.

While many in the transplant community have been critical of the President's duplicity, they could not deny that it was consistent with his basic philosophy that voluntarism and individual generosity are the way to solve social problems, not government intervention. Nor could they deny that with his unabashed showmanship, the President had raised some public consciouness about organ donation.

ACT TWO

Still operating out of Arlington, Virginia, the American Council on Transplantation sponsors a couple of sparsely attended transplantation conferences every year, puts out a fairly useful newsletter, and helps the families of transplant patients through the assorted bureaucratic mazes they face when a relative is diagnosed with organ failure. ACT is now funded primarily with membership dues from other national organizations and generous grants from the Sandoz Chemical Company (manufacturer of cyclosporine) and the Dow Chemical Company, which has no apparent economic interest in organ transplantation.

The powerful American Society of Transplant Surgeons (ASTS)—which, after Salvatierra resigned, publicly refused to join the federation—recently signed up and paid its ACT dues. Such an endorsement from the powerful brotherhood of surgeons greatly enhanced the prestige and independence of ACT.

Lack of prestige was something transplant surgeons understood. Until recent years they were barely recognized in either the medical or the surgical community as representatives of a legitimate or important specialty. Not until 1986, in fact, did the influential College of American Surgeons include transplantation as a recognized surgical practice or recognize the ASTS as a member organization. These attitudes simply reflected the degree of acceptance transplanters felt inside the large medical institutions where they practiced. And it's still not a love story either. "Sometimes we definitely feel like second-class citizens here," says Nick Feduska of his workplace.

Although professional respect for transplantation has improved markedly in the medical community, there is residual resentment in hospitals from the days when transplant units would suddenly occupy scarce operating rooms as others with less urgent patients were preparing for surgery; overload ICUs with very sick patients; flood laboratories with esoteric tests; overwork nurses; and put the institution at risk by accepting financially unstable patients.

CENTER PROLIFERATION

Today, hospitals have learned to live with transplanters. In fact, they all want into the transplant business. It's dramatic, lucrative, and adds a special prestige to any medical center that offers the service. What was Pittsburgh, after all, before transplantation? Just another decent medical school.

"Hospitals feel that if they don't have a transplant program, they can't be considered first-class," Harvard University health policy specialist Marc Roberts told the *Wall Street Journal*. "It's the new public works project. Everybody wants one." Even hospitals in communities with existing transplant units with long waiting lists and chronic organ scarcity seem eager to start their own programs. Perhaps they notice that hospitals with transplant services attract patients who don't need transplants. "It has become a marketing tool," according to Dr. Robert Corry, a former president of the ASTS. "If the public sees you are doing transplants, they are more likely to come in for their gallbladder operation because they have faith in you. You will also be more likely to have more success recruiting staff for all areas because they will want to be at a dynamite center."

In addition, it has been found that any new and exciting medical technology enhances the morale of staff that are already at a medical center. New technologies bring with them career-advancing teaching and research opportunities in surgery, immunology, histology (tissue matching), intensive care, and pharmacology.

Chiefs of surgery see the glowing publicity a single transplant can bring to an institution. They study the economics and find that the most common transplants—kidneys—are virtually guaranteed by the federal End Stage Renal Disease Program, and that heart and most liver transplants are now covered by about 80% of the Blue Cross/Blue Shield groups and most of the major private carriers. In most states, Medicaid will even cover some heart and liver transplants at selected centers.

Hospital administrators are constantly hearing directly from their physicians and surgeons about the number of patients that have to be referred out to transplant centers. Together, the administration and the chief of surgery take a proposal to their board, saying that it is time for their institution to move into the twentieth century. It's very compelling stuff and accounts for the rapid proliferation of transplant centers in the U.S. In 1978 there were less than 30 transplant centers in U.S.; by 1988 there were 226, and many more under proposal. In the long run, however, center proliferation may not be the way that transplantation expands. Existing transplant units are threatened by it and are beginning to present strong opposition to new centers opening in their regions.

When Fairfax Hospital, a private medical center in suburban Virginia, decided to open a heart transplant unit in 1986, its application was opposed by the local health planning agency which argued that Johns Hopkins, in Baltimore, and the Medical College of Virginia Hospitals were already providing adequate heart transplantation to the region. Fairfax appealed to the state commission. It took the testimony of impressive expert witnesses like Christiaan Barnard to get the proposal approved.

A similar conflict occurred in Pittsburgh, where a Certificate of Need (CON) for a kidney transplant center filed by Allegheny General Hospital was opposed by the University of Pittsburgh. Allegheny argued in its review that although the university did a lot of kidney transplants, its service was limited because it refused to transplant kidneys from living related donors. Although that wasn't literally true (Pittsburgh had done one such transplant the year before), chief of transplantation Tom Starzl did, and still does, strongly oppose the practice. Due partly to that fact, Allegheny's CON was approved. Starzl, whose center is still the largest in the world, has since complained about "the hyperplasia of centers," which, he says, has done nothing but "create a tremendous demand for organs."

When Santa Rosa Memorial Hospital, north of San Francisco, decided to offer kidney transplantation to its adult patients, the larger transplant units in the region politely wished them good luck. But privately the University of California, San Francisco, and others bemoaned the creation of another institution that would be taking organs from the pool. "They argue that they are serving their community," said one UCSF surgeon who asked not to be quoted by name. "Well, that's ridiculous. People drive from Santa Rosa to San Francisco to have lunch. They'll certainly come that far to get a transplant, and when they do they will be treated by a team that has done three thousand rather than a team that has done twelve. Take your pick."

Olga Jonasson, a Chicago cardiac surgeon who chaired the National Task Force on Organ Transplantation, which opposed the proliferation of smaller centers, says, "The cost of unnecessary duplication of expensive staff and resources is very high." But a more serious consideration, according to Jonasson, derives from the fact that the supply of organ donors is finite. "Every organ used in unqualified centers," she alleges, "is an organ transplant denied to a recipient in a qualified center where the outcome is likely to be better and where new and improved treatments are developed and available." Jonasson and her peers on the Task Force believe that strict criteria should be set and regulated before any new transplant center can be opened. An approved heart unit, for example, should be required to perform at least twelve heart transplants a year. For livers the recommendation was fifteen a year.

Christiaan Barnard, whose arthritis has forced him to retire from transplanting, now works as scientist-in-residence at the Baptist Medical Center of Oklahoma. He thinks the "centers of excellence" approach is "a lot of bull. Centers doing a small number of transplants can look after their patients." When he isn't promoting antiwrinkle creams, Barnard consults for the Baptist Medical Center's fledgling Transplant Institute.

The "centers of excellence" scheme does, however, appeal to the Department of Health and Human Services (HHS), which, a year after the Task Force recommendation, announced that

Medicare would cover only heart transplants done in centers that perform twelve or more transplants a year and have a one-year survival rate of 73% and a two-year survival rate of 65%. At the time, there were seventy-one heart transplant centers in the U.S. and only twenty met those criteria. Today, there are almost a hundred heart transplant centers and many more under consideration.

Private health insurance carriers and the Blues are following the HHS lead and proposing strict criteria for coverage. If they do apply strict criteria, it seems certain that independent procurement agencies will abide by the same guidelines and send donor hearts only to qualified centers, thereby driving more than seventy hospitals out of the heart transplant business.

Sen. Orrin Hatch (R-Utah), who authored one of the transplant bills that was eventually melded into the Gore bill, believes that setting criteria for transplant centers is "absolutely ridiculous. Why should the federal government give centers antitrust immunities by granting franchises?" he asks.

Roger Evans, a research scientist from the Battelle Memorial Institute in Seattle who studies transplantation economics and ethics for federal agencies and sat on the National Task Force on Organ Transplantation, believes that regional cooperation is the only thing that will preserve transplantation in this country. Competition for scarce organs in a restricted geographical area will result, says Evans, in fewer transplants being done at every center and will ultimately diminish the experience and expertise at all centers. "The more actors that become involved," says Evans, "the more complicated it will become from a distributional standpoint."

Norman Shumway cautions that smaller centers are not equipped to follow up patients on a long-term basis or to deal with the complications that often don't appear for years after a transplant. "Hospitals will use transplants as loss leaders," he fears, "hoping that the notoriety will bring them other kinds of cardiac surgery." Stuart Jamieson, now president of the Inter-

national Transplant Society, is more blunt. He says that proliferation of transplant centers is "wrong and dangerous, and the
net effect will be that more patients die."

Although these arguments contradict Orrin Hatch's concept
of free-enterprise medicine, they are nevertheless compelling to
most of the policymakers who impact and influence transplantation. As the surgery becomes more sophisticated, organ procurement more centralized, and the adjacent sciences of
immunology and tissue matching more complex, it seems certain
that human organ transplantation will become more and more
concentrated in large teaching hospitals like those at the Universities of Pittsburgh, Minnesota, and California, leaving the
smaller private hospitals to handle relatively mundane procedures
like open-heart surgery, kidney dialysis, diagnostics, and referral
of people with end-stage organ diseases to large transplant centers.

A creative solution to the proliferation crisis materialized in
Boston, where the Harvard-affiliated Brigham and Women's Hospital, with its successful heart transplant center, entered a consortium with three other local hospitals to offer a combined
transplantation service. The four hospitals agreed to share doctors, organs, operating rooms, support staff, and postoperative
patient care. While suspicious critics claim that the consortium
is something of a political charade designed to assuage local
officials while bringing more hospitals into the transplant business, the four Boston hospitals do appear to cooperate well in
the sharing of organs. If for no other reason, the Boston model
is worth observing as a possible model for regional management
of multiple transplant units. In fact, Boston can be compared
to Chicago, where there are also, coincidentally, four heart and
liver transplant units that are *not* operating in a consortium,
although in deference to the new UNOS regulations, they are
sharing organs. The state of Ohio is currently the only other
region of the country experimenting with a Boston-type system
that involves sharing patients, surgeons, and facilities along with
organs.

THE MATTER OF POLICY

Buried deep in the footnotes of reports gathering dust on the shelves of our bureaucracies, commissions, think tanks, and legislatures are answers to the truly tough questions raised by health policy analysts, medical economists, and ad hoc task forces— questions such as: Does organ transplantation really contribute to public health? Can government afford to support it? Where does it fit on the spectrum of healthcare priorities? Does the funding of transplantation favor the few who are very sick over the many who are not quite so sick or over the majority who are well but need protection from disease? Should we build transplant clinics or well-baby clinics? Should we build B-1 bombers or transplant livers?

Most of the equations used to answer these questions are well thought out, even mathematically sound at times. But they are incredibly complex. And no matter how much time analysts spend on their calculations, it remains so much easier for the rest of us to envision and appreciate the drama of one heart transplant than it is to envision and appreciate a million people not having polio. In the end, it seems, our legislators, bureaucrats, and independent commissioners are subject to the same sentiments. So most of the equations stay on the shelf.

In 1950 healthcare consumed 4.5% of the American GNP. By 1985 that figure had more than doubled to 9.4%. The 1988 estimate was close to 12%. As health costs continue to outpace economic productivity, and resource allocation is forced upon us, it seems certain that expensive curative technologies will be called to task more frequently by cost-benefit analysts and the decision makers they serve. The congressional Office of Technology Assessment found in a study that new medical advances (drugs, diagnostic machines, and transplant surgery) accounted for nearly one-third of the increase in Medicare costs over the past five years.

With statistics like that before us, should we proceed with

the publicly supported development of a completely implantable artificial heart, a device with unimpressive results that has already cost taxpayers hundreds of millions in research dollars? Should we support or grant tax advantages to firms manufacturing "orphan" drugs (very expensive treatments for very rare diseases) before research is funded for common diseases and epidemics? And more germane to transplantation, are we as a nation willing to grant to victims of any other ailment the same support we have granted to people with end-stage kidney disease—free dialysis or a free kidney transplant?

Since there is one factor common to all technologies—money—it tends to be the one used by most analysts. Studies by the Battelle Memorial Institute and other think tanks have actually demonstrated real cost-effectiveness for some transplants—particularly kidneys, which, two years post-transplant and even with expensive immunosuppression, show marked savings over dialysis, and heart transplants, which in most cases are actually cheaper than the postcardiac-crisis dying process.

However, no studies have yet been done that compare the cost-effectiveness of a dollar spent on a transplant versus the same dollar spent preventing the organ disease that necessitated the transplant. Some planners feel that the economic benefits of transplantation must ultimately be weighed against the costs and benefits of all other aspects of healthcare, such as prenatal care (which shows an almost immediate $2 to $3 return for every dollar invested), the prevention of birth defects (which affect 300,000 babies a year and create a vast population of people who sooner or later become dependent on the healthcare system), or the search for a vaccine against existing epidemics.

Those who will make the final judgment on transplant policy—government planners, insurance underwriters, politicians, and organ donors—must first consider its one unique quality. The major resource requirement is biological and finite. Other healing technologies that compete for the healthcare dollar are limited only by economics. With enough money, the supply of mechanical implants, pharmaceuticals, hospital wings, nursing homes, and well-baby clinics are theoretically limitless. No amount of money, on the other hand, seems to alter the supply of organs. Transplantation is therefore completely dependent on the voluntarism and generosity of the general public, without whose compliance there will be no organs to transplant.

It seems certain that within the next ten years health policymakers will conclude that transplantation can really survive only if it remains available to anyone who might, under different circumstances, donate an organ. Transplanters will have no alternative, it seems, than to advocate at least a partial socialization of their practice.

The groundwork for such a policy was laid by the 1986 National Task Force on Organ Transplantation, members of which were appointed by the Reagan administration. The Task Force adopted the position that "organs are donated in a spirit of altruism . . . and [therefore] constitute a national resource to be used for the public good." Following from that logic, Task Force members, only a bare majority of whom were transplanters, unanimously recommended that a "patient's financial status should not limit the availability of this medical treatment. All transplant procedures recognized as medically effective should be made available through reimbursement by existing public and private insurers. And the federal government should develop reimbursement mechanisms for the care of patients who have no other source of funds."

The Task Force's proposal reminds every policymaker with even a medium-length memory of the 1973 estimate of less than $200 million a year for the End Stage Renal Disease Program, which entitled any American who needed it to free dialysis. The program now costs Medicare close to $3 billion a year.

Conservative economists and health planners alike fear that soon after a Task Force–type policy is implemented, the demand for transplants will explode and the health budget will be ravaged. They point to the potential growth of pancreas transplants. There are 1 million insulin-dependent diabetics in the U.S. who could benefit from new pancreases. Unlike hearts or livers, pancreases can be transplanted (partially) from living related donors, obviating the need for brain-dead cadavers and organ procurement agencies. There is, therefore, an almost unlimited supply. If pancreas transplants (like kidney transplants) were to become an entitlement, at about $100,000 per transplant (the current average cost) the government would be looking at a $100 billion appropriation to cure existing diabetics. Planners also expect that shortly after transplants are given entitlement, neurosurgeons, cardiologists, oncologists, and pediatricians will be lined up for blanket coverage of their favorite life-saving technologies.

CHAPTER 11

WHAT NEXT?

The underlying premise of [our] technology is that nature can be understood and imitated.
Annual Report,
Organogenesis Inc.

The future of organ and tissue transplantation promises to be even more dramatic than its past. Like so many other biotechnologies, transplantation still awaits its major scientific breakthrough—something like cyclosporine, but on a grander scale. Once it comes, whatever it is, the development of transplantation will be exponential and a new concept of healing may well be established.

Transplantation's epiphany will probably occur sometime in the 1990s. With restricted funding for medical research, however, we may have to wait until the early twenty-first century, by which time science may have found cures for many of the end-stage organ diseases that necessitate transplants. On the other hand, another immunology pioneer like Peter Medawar may appear and, without government funding, find the key to immune tolerance, long-term cellular preservation, or an artificial organ that works. Failing those scenarios, the ultimate advance might spring from the massive gene-mapping project now under way at Lawrence Berkeley Laboratory.

Whatever the final outcome for transplantation, here are some near-term developments of which one can be fairly certain.

Medical scientists will eventually discover how to
induce immunological tolerance of specific antigens.

Selective tolerance, the ability to suppress only those anti-bodies that will attack a specific antigen, is the ultimate dream of transplanters. It will not come easily, as a billion years of evolution militate against it. But on the way to inducing tolerance, there will be preliminary developments worth mentioning. For example, according to Marvin Garovoy, chief immunologist at UCSF, it may soon be possible to alter the genetic structure of an organ during the ischemic period (when it is in between donor and recipient) so that it becomes either tissue-compatible with its new host or, better yet, a "naked organ" that will adapt to any immune environment. This alteration will be done as "bench-work," an operation performed on the organ itself after it is removed from its preservation solution and before it is implanted in its new host.

Attempts are still being made to induce tolerance in the host with radiation and bone marrow transplants although it is felt by most transplanters that the answer must be found in less radical technologies. Perhaps more promising is the work already being done on the prenatal manipulation of the immune system. In the 1950s Sir Peter Medawar discovered that when a fetus (Mouse A) was injected, in utero, with cells from an animal already born (Mouse B), Mouse A, when born, would not reject tissue transplants from Mouse B.

Dr. Leonard Bailey of Loma Linda University Medical Center, east of Los Angeles, now wants to try the same experiment with humans. Bailey's chief immunologist, Sandra Nehlsen-Cannarella, who trained under Medawar before he died in London, has convinced Bailey it will work. "As soon we know that a child will be born with hypoplastic left heart syndrome," says Bailey, "we can inject him or her, in utero, with cells from a donor [baboon or human] and, if Medawar's findings with mice apply to humans, the newborn should accept a heart from the donor without immunosuppression."

While transplanters wait patiently for induced tolerance, we can expect some remarkable breakthroughs in pharmaceutical immunology (some of them spillovers from AIDS research, others a continuation of transplant research) that will vastly improve both survival rates and the quality of life for transplant patients.

New Japanese "506" drugs may prove to be the next generation of immunosuppressants. Although they have already shown themselves to be imperfect in many ways, transplanters recall that early findings on cyclosporine were no less discouraging.

Monoclonal antibodies, new antilymphocyte sera, and steroids will also be prescribed in imaginative new combinations. And the quest will continue with cyclosporine, which itself can be greatly improved. But the next generation of immunosuppressants will probably not be as enthusiastically heralded as cyclosporine was unless the drugs are far less complicated or toxic.

The combined transplants of the heart and lungs, heart and liver, liver and kidney, kidney and pancreas may well become commonplace and lead to an era of simultaneous multiple-organ transplants.

Virtually impossible before the cyclosporine era, heart-lung transplants become more common every year as previously insurmountable hurdles are effectively addressed. Ironically, it is much simpler to transplant a heart and lung together than to do either heart or lung alone. The challenge arises in the pre- and postoperative vulnerability of the combined unit. It is also extremely difficult to preserve the two organs between donor and recipient, and rejection happens pari passu (together, at an equal rate). Combined organ transplants—heart and kidney, kidney and liver, kidney and pancreas, and in rarer cases combinations of three or more at once, even involving the bowel—have all been tried, with discouraging results. But as has happened with single-organ transplants, survival rates will undoubtedly improve in time, and multiples will become increasingly common.

The successful simultaneous transplant of heart, lungs, and liver performed in December of 1986 by Sir Roy Calne and Dr. John Wallwork at Papworth Hospital near Cambridge, England, showed that almost any combination was possible. The amazing "domino transplant," wherein the heart and lungs of a brain-dead donor were transplanted into a patient with pulmonary hypertension, who in turn donated his healthy heart to a third patient dying of heart failure, was first performed in April of 1987 by Dr. Magdi Yacoub of Harefield Hospital in England and repeated shortly thereafter at Johns Hopkins in Baltimore.

In November of 1987 the University of Pittsburgh did Yacoub one better by transplanting five separate organs into one patient, Tabatha Foster, a nine-year-old girl who in one operation received a new liver, pancreas, stomach, section of the large intestine, and colon. Although Foster died six months after her transplants, Pittsburgh's pioneering transplanter, Thomas Starzl, now claims to be ready, under the right circumstances, to transplant an entire gastrointestinal tract.

Lung transplants, which have been tried, but rarely with success, could become a major treatment for several terminal diseases, perhaps even lung cancer.

Until 1987 "lung-alone" transplants were rarely attempted. For reasons that surgeons could not fathom, the anastomosis of the trachea (connection of the windpipe) seemed to fail every time. Then, in May of 1987, Dr. Joel Cooper of Toronto, Canada, announced that he had found the solution: wrap a small section of the omentum (the membrane that holds abdominal organs in place) transplanted from the recipient, not the donor, around the tracheal anastomosis and it will heal. At the time of his announcement, Cooper had succeeded with eleven of his patients.

That was a world record. His technique is now being tried at most major transplant centers and should be in common use by the end of the decade.

Transplants of lungs alone will heighten one of the most vexing ethical dilemmas of transplantation. Should patients whose illness is caused or exacerbated by self-destructive habits, like smoking tobacco or abusing alcohol, be given scarce organs?

Bone marrow transplants will become a much simpler, less expensive, and more widely employed treatment.

Bone marrow transplants are currently used to treat several uncommon but extremely serious conditions, such as myelogenous leukemia, severe aplastic anemia, radiation poisoning, combined immune deficiencies, and some forms of Hodgkin's disease. Although an extremely simple surgical procedure, bone marrow transplants are immunologically the most complex and expensive of all transplants (easily running over $200,000 a case), due to the intense postoperative care that is required.

What is transplanted is not an organ per se but a conglomerate of stem cells that are responsible for the production of different blood cells. The transplant involves removing bone marrow from the donor's pelvis or sternum with a large syringe and injecting it directly into a recipient's veins (often following total body radiation). The stem cells find their way into the new host's bone marrow, and if all goes well, in four or five weeks the condition is healed. The transplant is complicated because bone marrow makes antibodies, and thus implanted marrow can create antibodies that roam through the recipient's blood stream, attacking the patient whom the operation is meant to save—usually someone whose own immune system is ineffective. The resulting chaos is termed graft-versus-host disease.

Almost any healthy living human being can become a bone marrow donor. Extracting the marrow is almost as painless as drawing blood and the donated marrow completely regenerates itself in a few days. The procedure may become even simpler when the technology is developed to spin stem cells out of regular blood. At that point, any blood donor could become a bone marrow donor. That is where the simplicity ends, however. While there are only four types of blood—A, B, AB, and O—there are literally thousands of tissue types. And with bone marrow, unlike some solid organs, tissue matching must be precise or the host will reject the marrow and die. About 1 in every 10,000 nonsiblings is a suitable bone marrow donor for any particular patient. With those odds, finding a match is a major challenge.

Most bone marrow transplants are done between siblings, where the chances of a good match are infinitely better than with donors from the general population. Even with donors whose tissue types are identical, major problems can follow, including rejection of the graft, graft-versus-host disease, or infection. Graft-versus-host disease occurs in about 70% of bone marrow transplants and ends lethally between 20% and 30% of the time. To protect against infection, the recipient is kept in isolation and fed massive doses of antibiotics for four weeks.

Bone marrow registries are now being formed to facilitate nationwide matching. The largest registry has been organized by the U.S. Navy, which would become a major end user of bone marrow in the event of a nuclear accident onboard a submarine or modern warship.

Pancreases will be transplanted as often as kidneys and become the treatment of choice for Type 1 (insulin-dependent) diabetes.

The pancreas produces trypsin, amylase, lipase, glucose and its inhibitor, insulin, along with about thirty-two ounces per day of alkaline juices that neutralize acid in the large intestine before it descends to corrode the small intestine. Yet this delicate three-ounce organ, about the size and shape of a dog's tongue, is so delicate that it cannot be touched by human hands during transplantation.

Pancreas transplanters debate among themselves more than other organ specialists. Like their contemporaries, they argue over who should get organs, when it is best to transplant, the ideal minimum and maximum ages of recipients, and other issues common to all organs. But pancreas transplanters are also undecided whether it is better to transplant a whole pancreas (with or without the duodenum attached) taken from a cadaver, or half a pancreas ("segmental transplant") removed from either a cadaver or a living related donor, or simply to transplant 100 to 150,000 of the million or more islet of Langerhans (insulin-producing) cells from a healthy pancreas into the portal vein or under the skin of a sick patient. And it has yet to be determined whether it is best to establish exocrine drainage of excretions by joining the organ to the intestine or to the bladder, or simply to seal off this exocrine flow by injecting a plastic plug into the pancreatic duct.

As with kidney, heart, and liver recipients, the pancreas transplant patient will likely require a lifetime of immunosuppression, usually involving the triple combination of cyclosporine, azathioprine, and prednisone. The most challenging postoperative problem facing pancreas transplanters has been the difficulty in detecting and treating rejection. Often the rejection is "silent" and unaccompanied by fever. Contrary to other solid organs, a pancreas cannot undergo a biopsy without damage to its functions. Physicians have therefore had to rely on inconclusive immunological monitoring to watch for signs of rejection.

By the end of 1986 there had been approximately 1,000 pancreases transplanted in approximately seventy hospitals worldwide. The University of Minnesota is the world leader, with over three times the number of the next largest pancreas unit. It is there that Dr. David Sutherland keeps the international pancreas transplant registry. Looking at the 700 transplants done since 1983, Sutherland reports a one-year graft survival rate of only 45% worldwide. But survival rates for grafts and patients vary widely from center to center. "If we look at the results of institutions with the largest experience here in the U.S.," says Sutherland, "we see sixty percent graft and ninety percent survival rates. Our longest surviving graft is now nine and a half years." That is not good enough in everyone's estimation to move pancreas transplantation from experiment to treatment—that is, a procedure covered by the major medical insurance plans. But it is an immense and encouraging improvement over the results of five years ago.

Pancreas transplants can cost anywhere between $35,000 and $100,000 (not counting the $10,000 per year postoperative costs). They are currently covered by about twenty insurance companies, including eleven of the Blue Cross/Blue Shield regions. Other carriers make decisions on a case-by-case basis and can often be persuaded by physicians that it would be cost-beneficial for them to cover a pancreas transplant rather than pay for treatment of the devastating secondary stages of diabetes.

It seems that there is more disagreement among transplanters than among insurance executives whether or not pancreas transplants are a good idea. Transplanters of other organs point to the high complication and infection rates as well as shorter life spans, in pancreas recipients, and they ask whether it is medically sound to replace insulin with the far more toxic cyclosporine and prednisone. Pancreas transplanters acknowledge the risks and difficulties, but remind their peers that pancreas transplantation is on the same place in its learning curve that heart, liver, and kidney transplantation was ten years ago. They ask for the same patience granted other transplanters in the past.

There are currently about a million Type 1 diabetics in the U.S., and between 12,000 and 19,000 new cases appear every year. Most of them could soon become candidates for either islet-cell or whole-organ pancreas transplants. Since it will be decades, if ever, before there will be a sufficient supply of cadaver organs to meet that demand, it seems likely that most of the transplanted pancreases, at least for the next ten years or more, will be harvested from living donors. That alone should keep pancreas transplantation in the realm of high medical and bioethical controversy.

Before the end of the century, hands and other limbs will be transplanted as a matter of routine.

Dr. Bruce Cunningham at the University of Minnesota is currently waiting for the ideal situation to transplant a hand from a cadaver to a patient who has lost both his or her own hands in a serious accident. Cunningham, a distinguished plastic and reconstructive surgeon, has already replaced several hands severed from their owners (autografts) but has yet to replace a mangled hand with someone else's (allograft). He has, however, been practicing hand allografts with primates, and with good results. So has thirty-year-old Dr. Patricia Egerszegi at the Hospital for Sick Children in Toronto, Canada. One of them will probably be the first to perform the operation on a human being, although Egerszegi says she doesn't feel she is quite ready. "I would like to do one or two more practice operations with baboons," she says. "Then I would feel comfortable doing a human."

Transplanting a hand, whether on a primate or a human, whether an autograft or an allograft, is an incredibly complex task. Most of the work is microvascular surgery performed through a strong microscope. Not only must bone, skin, and tendons be grafted, but also veins, arteries, and nerves. Countless minute stitches must be sewn, some of them with almost invisible sutures. Egerszegi estimates that, without complications, the operation would last at least eighteen hours. And it would be weeks after the operation before surgeons would know if the nerves had regenerated. "And let's face it," says Egerszegi, "that's the only reason to do it—to give the patient sensation as well as motor skills." Artificial limbs now give almost as much motor control as a transplanted limb. But tactile and position sensation is probably something that can never be reproduced mechanically.

Add to the anatomical complexities all the obstacles of rejection and one has a real surgical challenge. As long as immuno-suppression is as toxic or as risky as it is today, there may not be an obvious benefit in transplanting a limb. Perhaps it would be preferable to have a mechanical hand and not have to deal with the side effects of immunosuppression. "And," says Egerszegi, "we still don't know the long-term effects of antirejection drugs. We might be giving people cancer. I would not feel comfortable advising someone to try a hand transplant without telling them they might die from it."

Artificial organs and tissues will become smaller and more affordable, and will work almost, but not quite, as well as their human counterparts.

The medical premise of "The Six Million Dollar Man," a popular science fiction TV series of the 1970s, moved further away from fiction and closer to fact during the years when the program was aired. The plot: An important espionage agent is badly injured in an explosion. His mangled body is pieced back together by a brilliant team of plastic surgeons, bioengineers, mechanics, and chemists, who create a semihuman machine that continues to serve the intelligence sector by using his built-in biomechanical devices to listen through brick walls, see into safes, outrun trains, and crush deadly weapons with his bare hands. His hands, you see, are actually powerful gripping machines cleverly covered with sensate human skin. It is never made clear exactly which portions of the new man remain real flesh and blood. The most intriguing episodes tended to be those where the hero was placed in emotionally challenging situations. Only then could we discern the remnants of humanity in the bionic man.

That the series had some basis in fact was in part due to the work of people like Willem Kolff, a Dutch-born medical engineer at the University of Utah's Institute for Biomedical Engineering and Division of Artificial Organs. Kolff invented the first kidney dialysis machine in 1945. He was lured to the university in 1967 by its president, James Fletcher (now head of NASA). Kolff's mandate was to create the world's leading bionic research center. The results have been revolutionary. Robert K. Jarvik, developer of the first artificial heart, was a Kolff protégé, as was Stephen Jacobsen, who developed a mechanical arm and hand similar to the Six Million Dollar Man's, one with functional thumb and fingers and manual dexterity approaching that of a real hand.

Kolff and the University of Utah have spawned over twenty small biomedical companies, all nestled against the scenic Wasatch Mountains of Utah in an area now known as Bionic Valley. Such companies as Symbion Inc., formed in 1976, have gone on to manufacture the Jarvik heart and the amazing cochlear (artificial middle ear) implant that restores hearing to the totally deaf. Also in Bionic Valley are Life Extenders Inc., which has developed artificial bladders and sphincters; Vascular International, which makes synthetic blood vessels, and others companies that make insulin-administering heart valves, fallopian tubes, and devices that bring sight to the blind and movement to the quadriplegic. Elsewhere in the country, laboratories and venturesome researchers are developing artificial spinal cords, blood, ligaments, lungs, and skin.

The quest to build artificial hearts provides an intriguing closeup of the bionics industry and its government sponsors, and shows why the advance of artificial organs may move slower in the future than hoped by Kolff and his fellow inventors.

Development of the totally implantable artificial heart (TIAH) began in earnest in the early 1960s. The TIAH was an infant of the bionic dream. One of its first supporters, the General Dynamics Corporation, predicted the annual implantation of 600,000 plutonium-fueled versions of the device, which would, they claimed, save most of the 700,000 Americans who die annually of heart failure. A firm contracted to perform studies projected a per-implant cost of only $10,000. Another predicted that all the people who lived so much longer (because a TIAH would last longer than the failing human version) would add $19 billion to the GNP during the artificial heart's first decade. None of the TIAH studies addressed the possible technical, social, or psychological problems.

Upon reviewing these studies, the National Heart Lung Institute forecast that for $40 million to $100 million the TIAH could be ready by 1970, and set Valentine's Day as a target date for the first implant. Congressman John Fogarty (D-R.I.) chairman of the House Subcommittee on Health Appropriations, was sold; he declared that every minute lost in starting the program was condemning innocent Americans to an early grave. In 1964 $581,000 was appropriated to start the artificial heart program.

Two hundred eighteen million dollars later—and after two decades of extensive research and a lot of optimistic pronouncements from the renamed National Heart, Lung and Blood Institute, which funded most of it—the best that doctors and engineers working together could come up with was a rather noisy, awkward air-driven pump made of Dacron, metal, Velcro, and graphite, placed in the chest and supported through six feet of thick tubing by 350 pounds of cumbersome external equipment. And this was not the work of amateurs. The brains behind the first and best of the new hearts (the Jarvik-5) was Dr. Willem Kolff. Because the Jarvik was not *totally* "implantable," the "I" was dropped from TIAH, and the device became a total artificial heart (TAH).

The bizarre, if not depressing, specter of thousands of human beings moving about society attached to machines twice their weight has prompted the mechanical heart's developers, still well funded by the National Institutes of Health, to work harder on their percutaneous (through the skin) port-a-pack model, a thirty-pound battery-driven device that will transmit magnetic energy through the skin to an internal ring that powers a totally implanted heart.

Portability, however, is not the major challenge of the artificial heart. Even with tremendous advances in plastics and other synthetic materials, designers have had difficulty finding an interior surface for the space-age heart that won't damage blood cells and form clots that dislodge themselves from the surface and migrate through the body, causing embolisms and the kinds of strokes that plagued the final days of Barney Clark and William Schroeder, two early recipients of the Jarvik-7. Theirs, in fact, has been the fate of the majority of the small number of people who have been accepted into the TAH experiment.

The somewhat miserable and widely publicized final days of Clark and Schroeder raised the age-old biomedical equation that balances the *value* of extended life against the *quality* of extended life. They also prompted most of the surgeons who had implanted permanent artificial hearts to publicly announce that they would wait for considerable improvements before doing so again—reminiscent of the early days of human heart transplantation, when most of the first 100 operations done after (and including) Christiaan Barnard's ended in failure.

The quality of life, even of patients who lived for a year or more with the TAH, has made it difficult for Dr. William De Vries of Humana Hospital in Louisville, Kentucky, to find appropriate patients willing to accept an artificial heart on a permanent basis. But even De Vries, the only American surgeon approved to try the procedure, does not seem to be in a big hurry to try it again, even though Robert Jarvik recently announced that his latest model appears, at least in animals, to have beat the clotting problem. Animals, for some reason, have always done better than humans with the TAH (perhaps because they don't know what's in them). Thus, most of the recent human research on the Jarvik-7, the Phoenix heart, and their competitors has been on their use as *temporary* implants—as a bridge to keep desperately ill cardiac patients alive for a few days until a human heart can be found.

But bridging with a Jarvik has created its own disputes in the transplant community. Like transplanting living related donors, bridging is enthusiastically practiced and defended at some centers, while forbidden at others. The University of Pittsburgh is the major bridging center in the American transplant community.

Under the guidance of Drs. Bart Griffith and Robert Hardesty, fifteen Jarviks had been implanted by mid-1987; all but one of the patients received human hearts after being bumped to the top of the queue. Eight of them were still alive by the end of 1987. Pittsburgh is proud of these results and promotes the practice in the local media. Stanford University and the University of Minnesota, the other two large transplant centers in the U.S., both have strict policies against bridging with mechanical hearts, even though both centers lose people who might live a little longer with the device.

"Once you take out a heart and drop it in a bucket, you can't go back," says Stuart Jamieson, head of Minnesota's heart transplant unit, "and once you start the practice and move everyone who receives a Jarvik to the top of the list, as you must, then eventually you end up only transplanting people on the device and no one gets a human heart unless they are so sick they had to be bridged." Not only that, Jamieson points out that "the one-year survival rate drops from ninety percent to fifty percent for patients who have been bridged"—which means that any center that bridges with Jarviks ends up wasting half of its human hearts. And in a world where organs are almost as precious as patients themselves, that is a serious consideration. Jamieson does bridge his critically ill patients either by implanting a much simpler left ventricular assist device or by temporarily transplanting the heart from an older donor, which can be replaced with a younger human heart when one becomes available.

To the question of moving patients to the top of a queue, Tom Chakurda, spokesman for the University of Pittsburgh, responds, "But they are already at the top of the queue, by virtue of being our sickest patients." Although Pittsburgh appears to have slowed down its bridging program, Chakurda defends his center's policy. "Physicians cannot dictate the supply of hearts available," he says. "Their job is to keep patients alive. When all other alternatives are exhausted, what choice do they have but to implant an artificial device if it's there?"

Even William De Vries worries about the fact that extremely ill cardiac patients will be given priority over those with a better chance of survival. "Should we use that precious commodity," he asks, referring of course to a real human heart, "on a person who has already had his chest walked all over?" Eric Rose, a heart transplanter at New York's Presbyterian Hospital, is also opposed to bridging with Jarviks. "We don't want to use our supply [of donor hearts] on patients whose results, statistics show, are borderline," he says.

With all the uncertainty surrounding the mechanical heart, the most difficult question involves the question of when to remove the human heart. If it is taken from someone whose disease is in its early stages, one might be sentencing that patient to a shorter or a more pain-ridden life than if his or her disease had been allowed to run its course. On the other hand, if the disease progresses too far, the patient may be so weak and debilitated that he or she is unable to withstand the shock of surgery, or may have sustained kidney failure or other physical damage caused by a weak heart.

The artificial heart developers and most of the doctors who test their invention have recently been driven into the private sector, where venture capital and more compliant institutional review boards allow them to move faster than they could working in university hospitals under federal grants. Although there remains some research funding for permanent hearts, the left ventricular assist devices, which have had better results, have found favor with the funding agencies. Unlike human heart transplantation, the artificial heart program will probably have to be funded privately for a while, and the devices may be available only to those who can afford them. But that may change. Since the technology was first developed with public money, someone will eventually argue that the technology should be available to the public.

It is interesting to note that during the twenty-odd years that the artificial heart has been under development, there has been only one broadly representative committee formed to review it. In 1972 and 1973 the Artificial Heart Assessment Panel was created by the National Heart Lung Institute and charged with "detailing the economic, ethical, legal, medical, psychiatric and social implications of a totally implantable artificial heart." The committee included two lawyers, two economists, three physicians (a psychiatrist, a cardiologist, and a heart-lung specialist), a sociologist, a political scientist, and a priest-ethicist. The panel foresaw many of the problems that have arisen with artificial hearts, but their observations were largely ignored, particularly one recommending that "a permanent, broadly interdisciplinary, and representative group of public members [be formed] to monitor further steps and to participate in the formulation of guidelines and policies of the artificial heart."

Review of the program, however, is largely in the hands of technicians and experts, with occasional token participation by the "soft" disciplines. Harold P. Green, a law professor at Georgetown University and chairman of the 1972 panel, says that "this probably reflects a judgment that the technological imperative should not be thwarted by the musings of those who are concerned with the broader social, ethical, and policy considerations."

But the most important question, still rarely taken into account by exuberant promoters of fabulous devices, is the quality of life they offer their recipients. It is now well known that Barney Clark asked his surgeon, William De Vries, why he was being kept alive. The well-documented strokes and thromboses suffered by subsequent Jarvik recipients has made it difficult to recruit volunteers for another try. "Most people [still] aren't aware of the problems that go along with these transplants," warns Roger Evans, a research sociologist at the Battelle Memorial Institute in Seattle. People who have received a new organ, whether human or artificial, says Evans, "don't live the life of a person who is perfectly normal. They live the life of a chronically ill person."

De Vries responds that his "patients had a better quality of life than they ever had with the disease. The quality-of-life debate goes on, with emphasis from people who really don't know what happened.'' He claims that the Jarviks he implanted have had "more success than any type of medical device in history." Unfortunately, when De Vries made that claim, none of his transplant patients were alive to offer *their* opinions on the matter.

Roger Evans recently performed a massive study on heart transplantation for the federal government. He estimated that while as many as 15,000 people could be saved every year by heart transplants, only 400 to 1,100 hearts become available in the same time period. There are higher estimates of available hearts than Battelle's, but none that come close to 15,000. Battelle's estimate appears to have been pretty close. In 1986 there were 1,002 heart transplants performed in the U.S., up from 719 the year before and the less than 50 in 1980. At the beginning of 1983 there were fewer than 10 hospitals in the U.S. that would perform a heart transplant; today, there are almost 100. But the proliferation of centers has only lengthened the waiting list. At any given time, there are now between 3,000 and 5,000 potential heart recipients in the U.S. About 400 of them will get hearts. The rest will die while new people are added to the waiting lists.

These numbers suggest that the market has peaked, and with the current statutory strictures on organ request, brain death, and organ distribution, there seems no sign of anything in the foreseeable future but a serious heart shortage. For this reason, research and development on artificial hearts continues, despite serious mechanical difficulties and questionable benefits (given the expenses involved).

Tremendous advances will be made in the highly controversial area of fetal organ and tissue transplantation.

Although its primary purpose is to provide human tissue for scientific and medical research, the National Disease Research

Interchange (NDRI) could fairly be considered an agent in the tissue-banking business and part of the transplant community. In fact NDRI president Leatrice Ducat sat on the 1986 National Task Force on Organ Transplantation. In 1987, just over a year after the Task Force completed its report, she and the NDRI were investigated by the National Institutes of Health for selling tissue that had allegedly been removed from aborted fetuses that had not been tested for brain death or properly declared dead.

The investigation, motivated by unsubstantiated charges leveled by Washington-based right-to-life activists, made a brief splash in the Washington papers, then subsided from public view. However, the whole issue of utilizing aborted or stillborn fetuses came closer to public consciousness. Whatever the purpose of harvesting organs or tissue from human fetuses, it's an explosive issue. Feelings run so deep that it is difficult to separate emotional arguments from the arguments about emotion.

Most of the medical research in fetal tissue has been done outside the U.S. At the Shanghai People's Hospital in China, for example, doctors have been treating Type 1 (insulin-dependent) diabetes since 1982 by transplanting fetal pancreatic (islet of Langerhans) cells. Patients there have reduced their insulin dependency anywhere from 30% to 100%.

At the Karolinska Institute in Sweden, researchers have been preparing to transplant dopamine-producing fetal brain cells directly into the brains of people with Parkinson's disease. Research with rats obtained improved results over the autografting of adrenal tissue, which in 1987 became an experimental human treatment for Parkinson's. Similar attempts are being made to alleviate, arrest, or cure Alzheimer's disease and Huntington's chorea with fetal brain cell transplants. And Dr. Michael Harrison at the University of California, San Francisco, suspects that fetal liver tissue may cure thalassemia, an uncommon but serious hereditary blood disorder. Liver cells removed from animal fetuses and placed in other animals have successfully produced enzymes in the host. If successful in humans, this relatively simple procedure could obviate a fair number of liver transplants, at least those indicated for severe enzyme deficiency.

Fetal tissue transplantation could, in fact, dwarf conventional solid-organ transplantation before the end of the century. Not only are there many more conditions that can be treated with fetal tissue, there are also 1.2 million fetuses aborted annually in the U.S. alone. Fetal tissue also has one distinct advantage over its adult counterpart: it is immunologically naive. Not until they are born and well on their way to childhood do humans develop the surface proteins on their cells that stimulate the host's immune system to reject organs. That means, at least theoretically, that ABO blood type should be the only important matching consideration with fetal tissue. Fetal tissue is also much less likely than adult tissue to stimulate graft-versus-host disease, where the healthy tissues of a transplant recipient are literally attacked by antibodies from the graft. And prenatal cells, particularly nerve cells, regenerate much faster than the same cells would a few days after birth.

The strongest resistance to the idea of routinely harvesting tissue from abortuses comes from advocates for the unborn. "People who kill these tiny developing babies, by virtue of the fact that they have done the killing, lose any moral right to use those tissues," declared Dr. John C. Willke of the National Right-to-Life Committee. Bone marrow transplanter Robert Gale of UCLA responds: "All of us that work in fetal research feel that if someone has decided to have an abortion and gives permission, it is all right to use that tissue to help someone else."

Pro-lifers fear, naturally enough, that women will feel more comfortable having abortions knowing that something good will come of them. They also worry that if fetal tissue becomes economically valuable, an international black market might develop and poor women everywhere would begin getting pregnant simply to sell their fetuses. At least one woman has already publicly announced her intention to grow a fetus until its brain cells are mature enough to be transplanted to her father, who is suffering from Alzheimer's disease. The only thing stopping the scheme is her intent to get pregnant with her father's sperm to assure a better tissue match. Such a pregnancy would, of course, be illegal. The rest would not be.

Concern has also been expressed that some scientists might sidestep whatever statutes are passed to curtail trade in fetuses by buying ova from young women, fertilizing them with sperm bought from college students (just as sperm banks do today), and farming the fetuses in vitro, simply to harvest tissue for transplantation.

Subhuman to human xenografting, the transplanting of organs from animals to humans, will become routine before the end of the twentieth century. And genetically altered primates may well be bred and farmed to provide organs for human transplantation.

One has to wonder whether Hippocrates, when he wrote that "extreme remedies are appropriate for extreme diseases," could possibly have anticipated the Baby Fae case.

When an infant, born with left ventricular heart syndrome and code-named Baby Fae, faced certain death at Loma Linda University Medical Center near San Bernardino, California, Dr. Leonard Bailey sacrificed a young baboon, removed its heart, and transplanted it to the dying child. The world was shocked, not only at what Bailey had done, but because he had evidently failed to make an adequate search for a human heart in his anxiety to perform the experiment. A baboon heart was not as histologically well matched with Baby Fae's as it might have been. Bailey had a one-year approval from his hospital's institutional review board to try the baboon transplant, the approval was about to run out, however, and he wanted to try it at least once. Baby Fae died in twenty-one days.

Debates in the medical community over the ethics and propriety of this operation seem likely to last well into the next century. It is also easy to predict that the content of the debate will continue to focus primarily on the rights and health of the humans rather than those of the animals involved, that the ethical discourse will revolve around the propriety of placing an animal organ in a human body rather than the sacrificing a healthy living animal to save a human.

Animal rights advocates still consider "Baby Fae" a watershed case. Their concern, as one would imagine, is primarily with "Goobers," the young baboon whose heart was used. Tom Regan, a professor of philosophy, wrote in the Hastings Center report shortly after the operation, "Surely no one will seriously suggest that it was a matter of indifference to Goobers whether she kept her heart or had it transplanted to another. Are we not yet ready to see that creatures such as baboons are alive, and have a life to live? Those people who seized her heart, even if they were motivated by their concern for Baby Fae, grievously violated Goobers' right to be treated with respect."

An incalculable number of animals—mostly dogs, cats, pigs, horses, rabbits, calves, goats, rats, mice, chimpanzees, baboons or other simians—have died for the advancement of transplantation. Leonard Bailey, who already has a small baboon farm in his hospital, says he respects animals and those concerned for their rights but says that he, along with other cardiac surgeons and pediatricians, are faced with either letting babies like little Fae die or sacrificing some lower form of life to save them. Bailey points out, as others have, that pigs have been sacrificed for years and their heart valves transplanted into human beings —with little, if any, protest from either animal rights advocates or religious leaders. There was something about Goobers that seemed to set them off.

Before the end of this century, transplanters may routinely (and legally) remove organs from living babies born with atrophied brains.

There are at least 1,000 babies born in the United States every year without a cerebral cortex. Estimates range as high as 3,500.

Another 1,000 are conceived but aborted in the third trimester after their terminal defect is discovered. They are called anencephalics, are easily diagnosed at birth, and almost as easily diagnosed with sonography during the second trimester of gestation. Their forehead, which ends just above the eyebrow and slopes directly to the nape of the neck, clearly indicates the lack of a cerebral cortex. Without a cerebral cortex they will never see, think, experience love, or, most neurologists believe, feel pain. The longest anencephalic life span on record is five and half months. Most, however, die in a few days. Their condition, of course, is incurable.

Anatomically, everything about anencephalics besides their upper brain is usually normal. Most of them are born with healthy little bodies complete with a beating heart, functioning liver, normal kidneys, and enough brain function to stimulate breathing. Their perfectly normal organs could restore to normalcy or save the lives of thousands of other babies born with less debilitating congenital defects—like hyperplastic left heart syndrome, with which 400 to 500 American babies are born every year. The problem with anencephalics is that they die a degenerative death, so that by the time their breathing stops, their organs are useless for transplantation.

When Gail and Greg Marell of Oakland, California, were told that they were going to give birth to an anencephalic girl that would die a few hours, maybe a few days, after birth, their first thought was to donate her organs. Their obstetrician, Ed Blumenstock, called Michael Harrison, a pediatric surgeon at the University of California, San Francisco. Blumenstock knew that if anyone could use the organs, Harrison could. He had for years been transplanting infant organs in animals and had told his peers that he was ready to try some of the minute and tricky procedures with human babies. Harrison is excited by his discovery that fetal organs actually grew faster than the organs already in place in infants until they caught up to the size they should be. He is convinced that he can save hundreds of human babies with organ transplantation. Although Harrison is America's leading advocate for harvesting the organs of anencephalics, he had to say no to Blumenstock. The practice is illegal.

Why, asks Harrison, Leonard Bailey, and a growing number of physicians who are beginning to support their position, should parents not be allowed to donate the organs of children who will live only a few hours and never, even for a second, experience love or cognition? Why waste their organs, asks the outspoken Harrison, when "each year four to five hundred infants die of lethal kidney disease, an additional four to five hundred have congenital heart diseases, and another five hundred suffer deadly liver failure?"

His peers in medicine answer in chorus with a majority of the country's bioethicists, religious leaders, lawyers, and politicians: Because they are alive. Harrison responds that they are actually "brain-absent," which he says is the essential equivalent of brain dead.

However, "brain death," which is now legal death in forty-two states of the union, stipulates that there be no "medulary" (brain stem) function. Any human beings that exhibit any brain function, in the form of spontaneous breathing, for example, are legally alive—and even if they have no cerebral cortex, they are legally living human beings. Opponents of harvesting the organs of anencephalic babies argue that either defining these infants as dead or making an exception for their condition, no matter how noble the purpose, will hasten the slide down the slippery slope to euthanasia. Alex Capron, the University of Southern California law professor who drafted what is now the most widely accepted definition of brain death, is not quite so apocalyptic, but he does believe that "right now we have a very bright line [the specific definition of brain death], and that line could disappear."

Harvesting anencephalics is another of those topics discussed quietly within medical chambers. Very few physicians would today say publicly what Michael Harrison said, but a lot of them wish Harrison would prevail. Minnesota's John Najarian, the first transplant surgeon ever to become chief of surgery in a major medical center, believes anencephalic babies should not be harvested.

"Impossible," he said, "they're not dead."

"But two members of your team are for it," I said.

"Who?" he asked. I couldn't tell if he was faking.

"Stuart Jamieson." Jamieson had told me so in an interview the evening before.

"Well, he's crazy," said Najarian nervously. "Jamieson still lives in Africa somewhere."

(Jamieson, who is originally from Rhodesia, is surprisingly outspoken in his advocacy of harvesting the organs of anencephalics. In fact, he takes credit for "lobbying" California State Senator Milton Marks to introduce the first anencephalic bill in an American state legislature. When Marks, at Jamieson's urging, introduced a bill that said newborn infants should be declared brain dead as soon as they were diagnosed anencephalic, it was met with so much confusion and hostility in the legislature that Marks withdrew the bill. Marks, who says he might reintroduce legislation either calling for a study of the situation or again defining anencephalics as "dead," says that no matter which approach he takes, his bill would apply *only* to anencephalics.)

"And who else here is for it?" asked the gruff and anxious Najarian.

"Your new ethicist, Arthur Caplan," I answered. Caplan, to whom I had spoken that very morning, was a little more cautious than Jamieson in his position; he was, after all, the recently hired head of Najarian's bioethics department. He was also more cognizant than Jamieson of the public's fear of involuntary euthanasia: "I think we have to be very careful about how we word any proposed legislation changing the status of anencephalics. If a statute is worded right, it will probably pass."

At that point Najarian moved off his rigid opposition. "Well, it *is* working in Europe. In a way I'd like to see it, but in a way I wouldn't. You'll have people lined up at the door while women are having their ultrasound. It would look very bad for the transplant community. I really don't think the laws are going to change. There are just too many strong-willed people in this country who will fight against it.''

Meanwhile, more and more parents, aware well in advance that their child will be born anencephalic, are following the example of the Marells and offering to donate their baby's organs. Some even carry the child to term for that purpose instead of aborting the pregnancy. However, whenever they publicly declare their intention to donate and the right-to-life lobby hears of it, a suit is filed and the parents invariably lose. The legal argument still prevails. The baby is alive. Removing its organs would be the "proximate cause of death," i.e., homicide.

The anencephalic controversy has gradually worked its way onto the open agenda of the transplant community, where it is more exposed to the general public. At a special conference on pediatric brain death sponsored by the American Council on Transplantation (ACT), held in Washington in March of 1987, the discussion quickly moved to anencephalics, despite the hope of the conference organizers that it wouldn't. The discussion was heated. Although the majority present seemed strongly opposed to harvesting organs from anencephalics, it was clear that their motivation was neither moral nor ethical. They simply feared that the public response to removing organs from babies that were not legally dead would not be worth the risk it would bear for organ donation from other sources.

In April of 1987, a month after the ACT conference, the *New England Journal of Medicine* (NEJM) published an article by a team of German surgeons from Wilhelms University in Münster, West Germany. The German team announced that they had performed three successful kidney transplants with organs removed from anencephalic babies that by American standards would be considered living. According to the physicians, these transplants were perfectly legal because courts in the Federal Republic of Germany had previously ruled that anencephalics, even those breathing spontaneously, were never alive because of the absence of brain development. Two things were notable about this event. First was the very fact that the normally conservative and very prestigious *NEJM* chose to publish what the editors must have known was an extremely radical position in the U.S. But of greater interest to transplanters was the fact reported by the German surgeons that extremely small organs, when transplanted into ten- and eleven-year-old children grew rapidly to the size they would normally have been had they been the child's own organs. This meant that organs from infants, perhaps even premature or spontaneously aborted infants, could be transplanted into much larger human beings and become functional much more quickly than had been assumed.

The German doctors ended their article with this proviso: "We object to relaxing the protection of fetuses with anomalies less devastating than anencephaly, and also to offering any financial gain to parents who might allow their anencephalic infants to be born as organ donors." That, of course, was no consolation to right-to-life advocates in Europe or America, who saw the actions at Münster as an already unacceptable relaxation of protection.

The case of Baby Paul brought the whole subject of harvesting organs and tissue from anencephalics even closer to public consciousness. In September of 1987 Paul Holc was diagnosed in utero as having hypoplastic left heart syndrome. He was due to be born sometime in late October. A fetal heart monitor revealed his condition. His mother, a resident of Vancouver, British Columbia, was referred to Dr. Leonard Bailey at Loma Linda University Medical Center near San Bernardino, California. Bailey was recommended because, despite the controversy surrounding his practice, he still had the best record in treating left heart hypoplasia with transplantation.

Bailey recommended that Alice Holc be prepared to return to Loma Linda at a moment's notice. In the meantime, he said, he would issue an alert in the organ procurement network for an infant heart with her baby's blood type. Should a heart become available, Bailey suggested, Holc should then agree to allow a Caesarian birth of her child, shortly after which Bailey would transplant the new heart into the new baby. Coincidentally, the first response to Bailey's call for a donor came from Canada, but across the country in London, Ontario.

Baby Gabrielle was born in Orillia, Ontario, not far from London, about two months after a group of Canadian transplant surgeons, ethicists, and pediatricians held a meeting in London similar to the one held in Washington in March. Unlike the Washington meeting, however, the declared agenda of the London gathering was harvesting organs from anencephalics. American bioethicist Arthur Caplan flew up from Minnesota to deliver the keynote paper, in which he recommended statutes to allow this harvesting. Also at the conference was Tim Frewen, chief of pediatrics at Children's Hospital in London, Ontario.

When Gabrielle's parents brought their dying baby to London a few weeks later and told Frewen that they wanted to donate her organs, the consensus of the conference was still fresh in his mind: "In the presence of consenting adults it is ethical to offer life support" to anencephalics so that their organs will not degenerate in the process of dying. Frewen placed Gabrielle on a respirator. And Frewen sensed that he was making history. "This was the first instance that an anencephalic infant was offered life support in terms of an active decision," he said. That was probably true only in North America. The Münster team had done the same thing.

For the next two days Frewen and his staff watched carefully as Baby Gabrielle's condition deteriorated. On Wednesday he performed an apnea test. The respirator was removed to determine if she could breathe spontaneously. If she could, she was legally still alive and would be returned to the ventilator. But she couldn't breathe. So Frewen then declared her dead, placed her back on the respirator, and checked the UNOS donor registry to see if there was a request for infant organs.

As Gabrielle's respirated, beating-heart cadaver was flown from London to Loma Linda, Alice Holc was on a plane from Vancouver. They arrived about the same time, and within hours Leonard Bailey had removed Paul Holc by Caesarian section and transplanted him with Gabrielle's healthy heart. That night Gabrielle's body was flown back to Canada for burial.

The case of Baby Paul and Baby Gabrielle will be the landmark anencephalic test for years to come, and the protocol of placing a newborn anencephalic onto a respirator at birth and waiting for spontaneous breathing to cease will no doubt become the transplanters way of complying with contemporary brain-death statutes. And Leonard Bailey, perhaps the most controversial transplant surgeon in the world, will remain an advocate for harvesting anencephalic organs. "Anencephalics are custom-made to save four or five lives," he told me over a fast lunch in the Loma Linda cafeteria. "We ought to have at them. To me the saddest thing about the Baby Gabrielle case is that three organs went to waste; both her kidneys and her liver."

Bailey says he hopes that Sen. Milton Marks will reintroduce his anencephalic bill in the California state legislature. Arthur Caplan, however, feels that such an approach has little hope of success in California or any other state and believes that New Jersey Assembly Bill 3367 has a much better chance. The bill reads in part:

A parent of an anencephalic infant, either prior to or upon birth of that infant, may submit to the attending physician or surgeon a written request for the donation of the body of that infant, or a part thereof, . . . to which the attending surgeon *shall* consent in writing if the requested donation is medically suitable for purpose and safety, and if one of the parents does not object to the donation, *regardless of whether the infant has sustained an irreversible cessation of circulatory or respiratory functions or an irreversible cessation of all functions of the brain stem.* (Emphasis added.)

If AB 3367 passes, neither standard medical brain-death criteria nor existing brain-death statutes will apply to anencephalics, and for the first time in American history, surgeons will, be free to harvest organs from a (legally) living human being.

AIDS will become a critical issue in transplantation.

"The implications of AIDS are so overwhelmingly serious that patients in high-risk groups such as homosexuals, intravenous drug abusers, and hemophiliacs should probably not be considered to receive transplants until an effective treatment for AIDS becomes available." That position received little opposition when it was first posited by Nicholas Feduska at the Eleventh Congress of the Transplant Society in Helsinki, Finland, on August 8, 1986. And, naturally enough, no one contested his opinion about donors stated in the same address. "Potential donors who are homosexual, intravenous drug users, or hemophiliacs should probably be routinely disqualified, regardless of their HIV serologic status."

About a year later Feduska and his colleagues at UCSF decided that they would no longer accept homosexuals or any high-risk AIDS group for transplantation. "The mandatory suppression of their immune system just makes them an untenable risk for transplantation. We would be wasting organs," said Feduska.

About the same time that the University of California was deliberating its position, a liver arrived at the University of Pittsburgh from a cadaver donor that had proved HIV (AIDS) positive in an enzyme-linked immunoabsorbent assay (ELISA) test. Chief transplant surgeon Tom Starzl was hoping to transplant the liver into a very sick comatose adult male. When he received the results of the ELISA, Starzl approached the patient's family and told them about the AIDS test. He also told them that their relative was very close to death and that this liver was probably his only chance of survival. The family gave Starzl permission to transplant.

PITTSBURGH SURGEON TRANSPLANTS AIDS-CONTAMINATED LIVER, blared the headlines and the local evening news. In a hastily called press conference, Starzl calmly explained that the patient's family was faced with a modern Hobson's choice. The patient could be allowed to die in a few hours or be given two to five years of life with a new liver that would probably then give him AIDS. When Starzl explained that the family had granted informed consent, the story died down somewhat. And when the results of a Western Blot test (a much more conclusive, but slower, AIDS test) showed that the ELISA test had been a false positive, the story disappeared from the media. But that didn't change the fact that Starzl had, for all intents and purposes, knowingly transplanted an HIV-positive organ into a patient. Within the transplant community the issue did not go away.

While there have been several cases of AIDS being inadvertently passed to a transplant patient, both in the United States and Europe, that was the first known instance of a deliberate transplant, one that was almost certain to end with an AIDS death, as the patient's immune system would already be suppressed by antirejection drugs. "Tom Starzl has probably never seen a patient die of AIDS," says San Francisco General's Dr. Larry Pitts. "Even if he had, he still won't have to treat the patient who does die of AIDS. He will get his survival statistic, without having to observe the consequences."

AIDS is a sensitive topic among surgeons and physicians, particularly those who are close to blood and other high-risk bodily fluids. At the Seventy-third Clinical Congress of the American College of Surgeons, held in October of 1987, the first topic before the general session was "Confronting AIDS." It was the same year that three American health workers had been afflicted with AIDS by handling or otherwise becoming exposed to contaminated blood, and about six weeks before the meeting, the first prominent American surgeon announced that he was giving up his specialty for fear of AIDS. The fear of AIDS among surgeons and health workers only confuses the fear of passing it on to patients with organs. Starzl seems to experience neither concern, saying that he would do it again with an HIV-positive liver and, furthermore, that he would knowingly give an HIV-negative organ to a patient who already had AIDS.

First human tissues and eventually human organs will be cloned and manufactured for transplantation.

In July of 1986 biologist Dr. Eugene Bell took early retirement from his professorship at the Massachusetts Institute of Technology (MIT) to become chairman of the board, president, and chief scientific officer of an advanced biotechnology firm he named Organogenesis Inc. Nine years earlier Bell had become a household word in America's burn units by fabricating a "living skin equivalent," real human skin grown in a petri dish from a few "committed" human cells. Although it is literally cloned from human skin cells (actually from discarded foreskins), Bell calls his product an "equivalent" because he has not yet found a way to clone sweat glands, hair follicles, and other components of the human dermis. Until he does so, he cannot call his product "skin," only "skin equivalent," without being accused of false advertising.

During his tenure at MIT, Bell also explored ways to manufacture other living tissues and organs from human cells and tissue matrix models, and like so many promising scientists before him, he gave up all the academic kudos and prestige to profit from his discoveries. Capitalized in December of 1986 with an $8,000,000 stock offering, Organogenesis is already delivering cloned skin and blood vessels to reconstructive surgeons and burn units throughout the United States. The blood vessels are actually marketed by Eli Lilly and Company, which Bell contracted to handle the task. Organogenesis will soon offer "bone equivalent" and other connective tissues cloned from human cells. In the near future the company also plans to launch a new product called "Living Endocrine Pancreas Equivalent," pancreatic tissue cloned from real human cells, which could be used to treat America's 1.5 million diabetics and eventually obviate most pancreas transplants.

Would it be possible sometime in the future to fabricate real kidneys, livers, and hearts? Yes, according to Organogenesis spokesman Douglas Billings. "Conceivably it could be applied to any tissue type. First, we have to figure out how to induce cell differentiation in some of the more complex cells that we are now unable to harvest and culture in their committed forms. But once we have accomplished that, we should be able to take a mass of liver cells, grow them in whatever size or shape we want, and place them where they can be vascularized in a human body." Dr. Bell actually accomplished a similar task in 1981 when, after performing a thyroidectomy on a mouse, he transplanted cloned thyroid cells into the animal, which grew a new, vascularized gland where the old one had been.

And, Billings adds, the new organs produced by his company will be immunologically naked. "They will exclude those cells in the immune system which cause the rejection response."

The human brain will not be transplanted.

When one considers the enormous physiological task of reconnecting all the arteries, veins, nerves, and vessels that flow to and from the human brain, it seems unlikely that it will ever be transplanted by itself. Grafting an entire head would actually be a much easier operation, as the complex cranial and occipital nerves would be kept intact and there would be far fewer blood vessels to sew. All that would need to be anastomosed would be the carotid artery, jugular veins, the trachea, the esophagus, a few tendons, and, most difficult of course, the spinal cord. Physicians have not been able to reconnect spinal cords successfully, although there is a lot of research being done now.

Before cranial transplants are attempted, there should probably be some clarification of exactly what is being done. If Mel Brooks's brain, for example, were placed into the body of Mikhail Baryshnikov, whom would we have before us—Mel Brooks, the most beautiful comedian in Hollywood, or Mikhail Baryshnikov, the funniest ballet dancer in New York? Would Baryshnikov recover from the operation, only to ruin his dancing career by eating too many blintzes, or would it be Brooks, destroying his reputation by flirting with nubile teenagers? Until there is an answer to the existential question, Who is the end product of brain transplantation, further research should probably not be considered. But what has been done is revealing.

Robert White, a neurosurgeon now working in Cleveland, Ohio, has devoted a good portion of his thirty-plus years in practice pumping blood through isolated primate brains and transplanting heads from one monkey to another—all with an aim toward one day transplanting a human brain. White's early papers on brain transplantation were published in mid-1960s editions of *Transplantation Proceedings*. "We actually had very good results with monkey and dog brains." says White, who is a bête noire of the animal rights movement. "Then people began asking some very sensible questions, including: 'Your metabolic studies look good, your brain waves look good, but how do we know this brain which you have perfused with blood and oxygen is doing all those good things that brains do . . . thinking, cognitating [sic], and all those wonderful things that brains do?'

"At that point we moved into a program called 'total body transplanting.' That, after all, is really what you are doing when you transplant a brain or a head. You are giving it a new body. It also isn't far from what transplant surgery is doing now. They strip all the organs from a cadaver and sew them in living people. Why not leave them intact and give them all to one person— total body transplant? And you wouldn't have to sew up a single cranial nerve. And you would have an individual who could see, hear, taste, smell; and with modern electronics they could even communicate directly with his friends, family, and the public."

White, who is a devout Roman Catholic, has held discussions about his research with two Popes, Paul VI and John Paul II, whom he calls "J.P. Two." What did the Popes think? "Well, I actually spent much more time talking about it with Paul the Sixth, who probably knows everything now, than with J.P., who is really much more interested in healthcare and health policy than with research. P. Six was very much interested in my work. He was very praiseworthy and very excited by it.''

And what does White think are the metaphysical consequences of brain or "full-body" transplanting? "According to my beliefs, the being is contained in the brain. The spirit is in the cortex with memory, thoughts, feelings, intellectual capacities, sentiments, personality, faith. A cephalic transplant would [therefore] be, to my way of thinking, the transfer and survival of consciousness . . . a graft of the soul.''

White *can* conceive of circumstances under which a surgeon might transplant a healthy working human body onto a living head. "Say you had a brilliant scientist who had been in an auto accident a few years ago and was paralyzed from the neck down—a quadriplegic who was contributing great things to the world, and that scientist contracted incurable cancer in his bodily organs. Why not give him a new body? Chances are he would still be paralyzed, but he would have a healthy body to keep his brain alive.'' And that, White believes, could be done.

Would he perform the operation if asked to do so?

"Why, certainly.''

CHAPTER 12

EXISTENTIAL FIRE

Are we violating God's plan for creation?
ROBERT VEATCH, PH.D
Georgetown University

Let us beware lest, in the conflict between man and nature, both should be the losers.
PROFESSOR JEAN HAMBURGER
Paris, France

Before commencing debate on any new technology, one must accept the probability that it will have an upside and a downside, that those who praise and support a system may be as right in their thinking as those who criticize and oppose it. It is possible, after all, for the same technology to heal or to destroy (radiation), to protect or to poison (herbicides), to cleanse or to pollute (solid-waste treatment), to enrich or to impoverish (industrial agriculture). The problem is that no side in the debate may be considering all aspects of the technology.

Here, then, are some of the bright and dark sides of human organ transplantation.

Bright: Transplantation has contributed more than perhaps any other medical technology to our

231

understanding of immunology and end-stage organ diseases.

By saving the lives of people with serious organ diseases, transplanters have learned much about how the diseases work, not only by observing the removed organ but also by studying the nature of the patient's recovery. Whether or not an old disease strikes a new organ, for example, tells us much about the etiology and locus of the disease itself.

By striving to induce tolerance and combat the rejection response, transplant scientists have discovered many hidden secrets of antibodies and the intricacies of human leukocyte antigens. Their discoveries have broadened our understanding of immunity and contributed to research in unrelated areas such as autoimmunity, AIDS, allergies, and cancer.

Dark: Transplantation encourages a mechanistic, antiholistic view of health and the human body.

By concentrating so much diagnostic and curative effort on single organs and diseases, highly specialized physicians tend to overlook or eschew holistic considerations and treatments. As replacing worn and damaged parts becomes a more successful and widely accepted treatment, there is a danger that medicine will de-emphasize less dramatic diseases and less dramatic cures. If it can be fixed with a transplant, a disease somehow takes on more importance or urgency than others that can be fixed or cured with less spectacular treatments. This phenomenon, of course, has already led to the questionable appropriation of scarce human and economic resources.

Bright: Transplant surgery has advanced all surgery.

New techniques of anastomosis, anesthesia, perioperative management, and postsurgical intensive care that have been developed by transplant surgeons have been applied throughout the surgical field to other procedures, operations, and technologies.

Dark: Transplantation exalts invasive surgery, perpetuates the "heroic rescue" approach to healing, and advances the "acute care" model of medicine.

As we become more enamored with the drama and excitement of transplant surgery, we come to accept invasive surgery as a natural way to deal with disease. The danger is that we will come to define healing as a series of heroic interventions rather than an art. The consequence will be fewer lives saved at much greater expense.

Bright: More than any other medical specialty, transplantation has brought the public into the bioethical debate as an active and vested participant.

Because transplantation relies so heavily on public generosity and participation (organ donation), its challenging ethical dilemmas have been drawn out of the inner sanctum of medicine and into the political arena. This can only enhance democratic processes and improve the public's ability to influence the direction of future biotechnologies.

Dark: Transplantation perpetuates vivisection.

Few technologies sacrifice as many, and such a wide variety of, animals in their research as transplantation. Transplanters claim there is no other way to develop their skill and knowledge than to practice and experiment on "lower life forms." Animal advocates say the carnage has been excessive and unnecessary, some even arguing that animal experimentation has retarded the progress of human transplantation.

Bright: Transplantation balances the animal rights debate.

Because the use of animals in transplant research is so much more humane than it is in so many other scientific experiments, and the purpose so much nobler, it is difficult for antivivisectionists to take an absolute position on animal research. Few of them have said, for example, that they would be happy having a relative operated on by a young surgeon, performing his first transplant, who had not practiced at least a few times on pigs or rabbits.

Dark: Transplantation has compromised society's respect for the dead.

We are beginning to see a "cadaver" less as the remains of a once living, laughing human being and more as a source of tissue—even an economic resource.

CARTESIAN TECHNOLOGY

Human organ transplanting is in some ways an inevitable end-product of the Newtonian era—a philosophical epoch beginning in the early eighteenth century that melded the world views of Sir Isaac Newton, René Descartes, and others; where nature came to be seen as raw material and man as machine. Once the temple or personal property of God, as it remains only in Islam, the human body has (with help from Descartes, Newton, and Darwin) joined the engine in the Western industrialized mind. Responsibility for the maintenance of nature, and with it the body, thus shifted from God to physician-scientist.

As we learned how to replace the worn parts of our engines, we strove to replace our own. And as with so many of our other technologies, we became so awed by our ability to transplant organs that we embraced the treatment before examining its metaphysical consequences. Only after organ transplanting was well established as a medical specialty did we invite philosophers and religious leaders to explore what it might mean to the future of the human condition. The peril of transplanting, they find, does not lie in its questionable healing powers. The danger lies in how we humans will come to see ourselves if replacing worn parts and damaged organs becomes the dominant paradigm of healing.

Will organ transplantation lead us to become, as prominent French transplanter Henri Kreis predicts, a sort of "patchwork man"—a passive-aggressive species so desperate for a little longevity that we willingly support an enormously expensive and ethically troubled technology, sacrificing the resources of public health, forgoing research in preventive medicine, even risking the loss of some major epidemiological battles in the process? Might we one day even compromise our deepest religious beliefs to serve the cause of organ procurement?

Not one nation in the European-American world has developed an effective democratic mechanism to study and challenge the application of emerging technologies. The very question, Should we apply this technology? is anathema to modern scientific inquiry. Those who raise it are branded heretics, neo-Luddites, or worse. Modern technoheretics, however, seem right about one thing: We are drawing close to the point where our faith in scientists working in corporate laboratories, universities, and hospitals is equal to our faith in God or nature.

It has only been within the last few years that leaders of the world's great religions have begun to ponder the ramifications of this tendency, particularly as it applies to organ transplantation. True, there had been those of Judaic or Christian persuasion who took positions on both sides of the brain-death issue. And there had been occasional outbursts of indignation from church leaders reacting to specific transplant events or practices. And European-American Christian ethicists had debated the moral implications of required request, presumed consent, the methods of selecting recipients for scarce organs, and the desecration of corpses. But even in Judeo-Christian societies, where most of the transplantation has taken place, there has been very little thought given to the impact of the technology itself on either the human condition or the human soul. Islamic and Buddhist leaders in the less developed world have barely given it a thought. And scholars of those faiths studying in the Western world can only fall back on semirelated ancient teachings to conjecture what people of their faith should think about transplanting organs.

ISLAM

Islamic scholar Abdulziz Sachedina lives in Canada and lectures at Haverford College in Pennsylvania. He says that with the emergence of Islamic fundamentalism, younger physicians in the Muslim world have become more concerned with the impact of Western medical practices on their faith. To Muslims, one's body is the property of God, not of the person. "We are merely stewards or trustees of our bodies," says Sachedina.

While the Koran teaches that resurrection involves the entire body, in Sachedina's opinion that does not preclude the donation and removal of organs, with one proviso—the recipient must assure the donor that he or she will never allow his or her body to be cremated with the donor's organ in it. Should a non-Muslim recipient (and it is acceptable to donate organs to people of other faiths) choose to be cremated, he or she must have the transplanted organ removed and buried separately before the body is burned.

BUDDHISM

American Buddhist leader Kenyu Tsuji says that, as in Islam, Buddhist leaders do not have an official position on organ donation or transplantation, and that there is very little in the fundamental dharma (teachings) of the great Roshis (teachers) that would create a position. The concept of bodhisattva places the welfare of others before one's own and encourages transfer of the self into the larger self, or, in Tsuji's words, "merging with the cosmic compassion of the universe.

"An enlightened view of the body and its relationship to the whole universe will immeasurably enhance the quality of human life. Donating organs so that other persons may live is indeed a noble act," says Tsuji, who is quick to point out that it is only his opinion. "In the realization of the oneness of mankind and the universe, human beings will share in the suffering as well as the happiness of their fellow human beings."

JUDAISM

When Christiaan Barnard performed the first heart transplant in 1967, orthodox Jews publicly condemned transplantation as "double murder." Today, after twenty years of reconsideration by rabbis and scholars of the faith, an organ donation is considered a mitzvah—a good deed.

There remains an ancient Jewish law called Kavod Hamet, which says that only intact bodies may enter the kingdom of heaven and that the soul is cognizant of the body's mutilations. However, according to Dr. David Weiss, an orthodox Jewish scholar in Jerusalem, Jews are not bound by any single ancient law but follow "the normative mainstream traditions of their faith, which is in a continuous process of unfolding." The Kavod Hamet is by no means "mainstream," nor is it binding on any but the most fundamentalist Jews. Not only is the transplantation of tissues and organs legal in today's Jewish faith, but "it is encouraged and mandated" says Weiss. "Jewish law is given to people as something to live by, not to die by."

It is true, he admits, that transplantation lessens the Jewish concept of man's inviolable wholeness. Jewish leaders, he says, have not yet decided "at what point the removal of a person's parts affects his individuality or the inviolable dignity of man's physical fabric. But we are in agreement, and have been for centuries, that the saving of human life overwhelms all other

considerations." Weiss cautions that the degree of risk to both
donor and recipient must at all times be taken into account. "One
may not lay down their life for anyone else or vice versa."

CHRISTIANITY

Since most transplanters have been Christians, it might follow
that Christian leaders would have given more thought and made
more specific pronouncements on transplantation than leaders of
the other religions. Not so. Christians have certainly wrestled
with some of the issues surrounding transplantation, but in in-
imitable Western fashion, they have accepted the technology as
if it were as much a gift of God as our bodies themselves. William
May, the noted Christian theologian and ethicist, traces our un-
challenging acceptance of transplantation and other high-tech
medical cures to the residual influence of the Gnostics, an early
Christian sect which, like its Hellenic counterparts, preached that
salvation came from knowledge (from the Greek *gnosis*, which
means knowledge).

It is Gnostic faith, says May, that led directly to the modern
reliance on professionals. "We look to the professional's knowl-
edge-based power to improve the world and its failing bodies,"
he says. "Technology, under this faith, tends to treat nature as
incidental raw material to be converted into miracle drugs and
wonder products. This general outlook, linked with the general
good intentions of modern technology, provides a spiritual basis
for the strategy of routine salvaging of organs and other material
from the body."

But May says that the religious optimism inherent in early
Christianity has been countered by a pessimism that "exists in
all religions. It is entirely unofficial in our society, yet it domi-
nates our culture. It is the pervasive modern conviction that the
powers that rule the universe are random, multiple, evil, and
destructive rather than nurturing, creative, and preservative. We

need look no further than the headlines of our daily newspapers. Explosive, destructive, arbitrary power makes the news. And modern medicine operates within this rather pessimistic understanding of the universe. "Disease," says May, has come to be seen as something that "results not from the withdrawal of a positive, life-giving power but from the invasion of a negative, destructive power. The germ theory has become the basic metaphor under which we interpret all disease.

"Healing, then, occurs not through the retrieval of a lost positive, the recovery of health, but rather through battle with an aggressive negative. Hence: 'The *war* against cancer, the *war* against heart disease, etc.' We have come to see ourselves as hostages to abusive and hostile powers and forces that will eventually do us in. Hence the drive behind the healthcare system to fight unconditionally against death. We seek to avoid death (hence the temptation of friends and staff to withhold the whole truth from the stricken and the dying).

"These two responses of resistance and avoidance create the crisis we face in organ donation. The strategy of resistance creates the demand for ever more organs and transplants to stave off death. But the reflex of avoidance makes it extremely difficult to get individuals to donate their organs to further that fight. Signing the donor card forces them to reckon with the fact that they will one day die. Thus, avoidance dodges what resistance demands."

May sees emerging in the Judeo-Christian world a third view that is neither optimistic nor pessimistic. It sees the body as real and affirms "a profound link in identity of the spirit with its somatic existence." Modern Judeo-Christians would not be so ready as the Gnostics to justify invasion of the body, living or dead, without explicit consent. "A person not only *has* a body, she *is* her body," says May. "So argued the Jewish and Christian existentialists of our time. While the body retains a recognizable form, even in death, it commands the respect of identity. No longer a human presence, it still reminds us of that presence which once was utterly inseparable from it."

With this in mind, Judeo-Christian society has bestowed quasi-property rights on a corpse to the family of the deceased ("quasi," in the sense that the cadaver cannot be used for commercial purposes). It is clearly this tradition that makes it impossible for transplanters to act on the letter of the Anatomical Gift Act and salvage organs simply because the deceased is carrying a signed donor card.

METAPHYSICAL FIRE

No longer pressed with the pace and tumult of heroic surgery, Jean Hamburger, the brilliant French nephrologist who performed what is arguably the first successful kidney transplant in the world, now ponders and writes about the impact of his chosen practice on man, medicine, science, and the universe. He is bright, effusive, formal, and meticulous, but like all great scientists, he is anxious that his views be heard and understood long after he is gone. There is barely room for two in his tiny office near the Sorbonne in Paris.

On November 17, 1947, Hamburger published his first paper on kidney transplants in dogs and on skin grafts in mice. In it he predicted the major problems that organ transplanters would face for the next forty years. He was mostly right. It would be decades, he said, before scientists would fathom and control the immune response. The most challenging reality that transplanters would face in the years to come would be the fact that while the immune system is basically similar among all mammals, it is completely different in structure from mouse to mouse, person to person. So even after we have discovered how immunity works, we will still be faced with the stubborn bioindividuality of humans.

"It is this magnificent difference," he reminds us, "that protects our species and has allowed us to evolve. If our immune systems were identical, we would have been annihilated millenniums ago." It is, ironically, the same mechanism that allows us to survive that now presents transplanters with such an enormous challenge. "Scientific irony," Hamburger calls it. "No [other] animal rebels against his destiny," the surgeon-philosopher writes of humanity in his classic essay "Discovering the Individual." "We never cease to express through behavior and language our rebellion against the contradiction between the world as it is and the world we dream of."

That organ transplantation has contributed enormously to the rest of medicine is, in Hamburger's mind, self-evident. It was the challenge of combating rejection, he says, that gave impetus to the new science of immunology and led to "our discovery of that strange army of cells that protect us from diseases that we don't even know exist, of interleukins and a host of other things whose import goes so far beyond transplantation. We also learned from our research that rejection of antigens is not a 'yes or no' phenomenon but a balance of forces for and against acceptance. And from transplantation we learned about the true nature of autoimmunity, which may contribute to as many as half of all human diseases."

In 1947 Hamburger did not predict that the transplantation era would end. Now he does. "The marvel of this story is that the advances in our understanding of [end-stage organ] diseases will have largely originated in studies of transplantation immunology. Understanding them, of course, will help us cure them. When we do, the era of transplantation will have engendered the possibility of avoiding transplantation."

But before transplantation becomes another brilliant episode in medical history, Hamburger says, we may suffer a natural backlash. "Natural law decrees that children born with a hereditary defect must die. This we feel is unfair. We ask medicine to right this wrong. And it does so. It is another victory in our struggle against nature, its injustices and cruelty. But in making these conquests man is playing with fire. Preventing the natural death of children with hereditary defects increases the defect when the patient matures, marries, and procreates."

Hamburger acknowledges that we began this process long ago in medicine, with the development of insulin and other maintenance medicines for phenylketonuria, hypertension, mental diseases, etc., but says that because we have done it before doesn't mean we can afford to do it forever. "Nature's schemes and mankind's dreams have different purposes," he says. "Yet pacific coexistence is necessary. It is necessary because nature might otherwise exact such severe penalties that all our successes would come to naught."

It is not common for surgeons and physicians to raise such prescient questions about medicine, particularly about their chosen specialty. But Hamburger is no common surgeon. Most transplanters, when approached with these topics, have either refused to deal with them or become quite defensive. "I'm afraid I am not in a position to respond to your rather sweeping philosophical propositions," wrote Francis D. Moore, medical historian and surgeon-in-chief emeritus at Boston's Peter Bent Brigham Hospital, in response to a letter seeking an opinion of Hamburger's theses. "Transplantation of organs has been reasonably successful in bringing relief of suffering to many very sick patients; as long as it does this job, society will continue to want this service," Moore said before closing his very polite letter.

John Najarian, chief of surgery at the University of Minnesota, was more defensive, particularly on the gene-pool question. "The genetically based diseases that we are treating with transplantation are in the minority," he said, seeming to miss Hamburger's point that treating them successfully could push genetic diseases into the majority.

Tom Starzl, who for better or worse is emerging as the dean of American transplanters, passes a warning to his colleagues similar to Hamburger's. "The consequences of changing human ecology are well known to those who have studied the amplifying effects of antibiotics on the population explosion that is said to threaten the earth or at least the quality of life of its inhabitants," says Starzl. "It remains now to be seen how society will manage transplantation, the most recent product of its creativity and sponsorship."